Handbook of Otolaryngic Allergy

Christine B. Franzese, MD, FAAOA
Professor of Clinical Otolaryngology
Director of Allergy
Department of Otolaryngology
University of Missouri Health Care
Columbia, Missouri

Cecelia C. Damask, DO
Clinical Assistant Professor
Department of Otolaryngology—Head and Neck Surgery
University of Central Florida
Orlando, Florida
Private Practitioner
Lake Mary Ear, Nose, Throat & Allergy
Lake Mary, Florida

Sarah K. Wise, MD, MSCR
Professor
Department of Otolaryngology—Head & Neck Surgery
Director
Residency Program
Emory University School of Medicine
Atlanta, Georgia

Matthew W. Ryan, MD
Associate Professor
Department of Otolaryngology—Head & Neck Surgery
UT Southwestern Medical Center
Dallas, Texas

72 illustrations

Thieme
New York • Stuttgart • Delhi • Rio de Janeiro

Acquisitions Editor: Timothy Hiscock
Managing Editor: Apoorva Gaurav Prabhuzantye
Director, Editorial Services: Mary Jo Casey
Production Editor: Rohit Dev Bhardwaj
International Production Director: Andreas Schabert
Editorial Director: Sue Hodgson
International Marketing Director: Fiona Henderson
International Sales Director: Louisa Turrell
Senior Vice President and Chief Operating
    Officer: Sarah Vanderbilt
President: Brian D. Scanlan

Library of Congress Cataloging-in-Publication Data
is available from the publisher

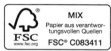

© 2019 Thieme. All rights reserved.

Thieme Publishers New York
333 Seventh Avenue, New York, NY 10001 USA
+1 800 782 3488, customerservice@thieme.com

Thieme Publishers Stuttgart
Rüdigerstrasse 14, 70469 Stuttgart, Germany
+49 [0]711 8931 421, customerservice@thieme.de

Thieme Publishers Delhi
A-12, Second Floor, Sector-2, Noida-201301
Uttar Pradesh, India
+91 120 45 566 00, customerservice@thieme.in

Thieme Publishers Rio de Janeiro,
Thieme Publicações Ltda.
Edifício Rodolpho de Paoli, 25º andar
Av. Nilo Peçanha, 50 – Sala 2508
Rio de Janeiro 20020-906 Brasil
+55 21 3172 2297

Cover design: Thieme Publishing Group
Typesetting by DiTech Process Solutions, India

Printed in Germany by CPI Books, Leck   5 4 3 2 1

ISBN 978-1-62623-906-7

Also available as an e-book:
eISBN 978-1-62623-907-4

Important note: Medicine is an ever-changing science undergoing continual development. Research and clinical experience are continually expanding our knowledge, in particular our knowledge of proper treatment and drug therapy. Insofar as this book mentions any dosage or application, readers may rest assured that the authors, editors, and publishers have made every effort to ensure that such references are in accordance with **the state of knowledge at the time of production of the book.**

Nevertheless, this does not involve, imply, or express any guarantee or responsibility on the part of the publishers in respect to any dosage instructions and forms of applications stated in the book. **Every user is requested to examine carefully** the manufacturers' leaflets accompanying each drug and to check, if necessary in consultation with a physician or specialist, whether the dosage schedules mentioned therein or the contraindications stated by the manufacturers differ from the statements made in the present book. Such examination is particularly important with drugs that are either rarely used or have been newly released on the market. Every dosage schedule or every form of application used is entirely at the user's own risk and responsibility. The authors and publishers request every user to report to the publishers any discrepancies or inaccuracies noticed. If errors in this work are found after publication, errata will be posted at www.thieme.com on the product description page.

Some of the product names, patents, and registered designs referred to in this book are in fact registered trademarks or proprietary names even though specific reference to this fact is not always made in the text. Therefore, the appearance of a name without designation as proprietary is not to be construed as a representation by the publisher that it is in the public domain.

To my husband, Michael, and my daughters, Catherine and Chrissy: Thank you for all your love, support,
and patience with me while I worked on this project. I could not have accomplished this without you.
Now, I can focus on what truly matters—spending time with my awesome family, playing Dungeons & Dragons, and cosplaying at Comic Cons.

To my coeditors, Sarah, Cecelia, and Matt: You guys are amazing. Thank you so much for your help.
This book would not have happened without you. Huzzah!

Christine B. Franzese

Contents

Contents

Foreword

This book has information-rich text supported by ample and recent references; therefore, it is much more than a "handbook." The list of contributors reflects the participation of most of the notable lecturers and researchers in the subspecialty.

The book benefits from the editors' caliber, as duplication of materials even in closely related chapters is kept to a minimum, thus saving the valuable time of readers. It is not a pedantic tome and tends to resemble the student-friendly approach of basic and advanced courses of the American Academy of Otolaryngic Allergy (AAOA). The text is supported by frequent use of "clinical pearl" and "how I do it" approaches. Even the basic science concepts are presented in the form of bullet points to emphasize the facts with most clinical relevance. Toward the end of the book there is a "practice makes perfect" section of clinical vignettes (and answers) involving critical techniques, such as assembling the starting, then maintaining immunotherapy vials based on an individual's skin or sIgE testing results.

The authors have included answers to most common questions posed by residents to the faculty at lectures. These questions include queries from our patients who venture outside the realm of fact-based medicine. Hence, there are short chapters on herbal/homeopathic remedies and acupuncture.

Many courses and virtually all articles fail to address the essentials for integrating otolaryngic allergy into a practice, but without these the clinicians waste time and resources. Yes, sometimes senior colleagues can direct you but they may not know the most up-to-date or efficient practices (which in my case took me years to realize). The editor recognizes the issue, so the final chapters of the book are devoted to the mechanics of setting up the office, selecting/training staff, patient selection, and billing/coding.

It has been nearly a decade since a comprehensive review on otolaryngic allergy has appeared, and this book was sorely needed for this, if for no other reason. The fact that it is succinct, well written, and highly clinician-friendly is a bonus. As with all books, no matter how comprehensive, the text does not abrogate the clinician's responsibility to periodically attend courses or an annual meeting to keep abreast of rapidly evolving topics or less common aspects of the subspecialty. That said, if one practices otolaryngic allergy, this book is currently the single best resource and should be within ready reach in the office.

J. David Osguthorpe, MD
Former Professor
Department of Otolaryngology—Head and Neck Surgery
College of Medicine
Medical University of South Carolina
Ralph H. Johnson VA Medical Center
Charleston, South Carolina

Preface

Congratulations reader! You have just made the best possible book purchase you could ever hope to make in your entire life with the money you spent on this book. Hopefully, you actually read the title of the book and have some passing interest in learning about the practice of allergy, but even if you couldn't care less about Type I IgE-Mediated Hypersensitivity, all is not lost! This book will fill a void in your soul that you didn't know existed. However, if you have no soul or aren't concerned about any holes in it, this book will give you loads of practical knowledge and useful tips that you can use in everyday allergy practice, whether you are a Total Noob in the World of AllergyCraft or a final level boss.

This book should soon become a well-worn companion to you, sitting close to you in your office or dwelling in your coat pocket. Its pages will shortly become dog-eared, its cover will become coffee and/or food stained. You might write in it, underline or highlight certain areas, or just gaze lovingly at its text. Listen, I don't judge. What you should not do is let this book sit on a shelf somewhere. That's an utter waste of your hard-earned dough, and if that's all you want to do, I have a much better suggestion! Take whatever amount of the said hard-earned dough you'd like to waste and send it to the University of Missouri, Columbia Department of Otolaryngology, ATTN: Christine Franzese, One Hospital Drive, Suite MA314, Columbia, MO 65212. No amount is too small (or too large!), and I accept all major credit cards or forms of currency.

On a [slightly] more serious note, the idea for this book blossomed from three issues I was having whenever I attempted to increase my knowledge base through the printed world. The first being that I would read all these wonderful, majestic tomes and manuscripts—encyclopedias filled with a wealth of background knowledge on allergic disorders and the practice of allergy—but when it was time to get to the good stuff—the actual how-do-you-really-do-it part—well, that was disappointingly missing. Instead of clear descriptions of what should be done, there were vague sentences that glossed over the actual testing procedure or protocol. Although I was wiser in foundation knowledge, I still was not sure how to put that knowledge into practice. The other issue was that the above-referenced wonderful, majestic tomes and manuscripts dripping with rich allergic knowledge (could that be mucus?) were also deadly boring. Don't get me wrong, they're fantastic reference material. But they also have a marked tendency to induce immediate, irresistible somnolence. I rapidly found I could not absorb knowledge into my brain by sleeping on the text. On that note, I did find that some of these articles did contain practical knowledge (I propped open my eyes with toothpicks to do this), but it took forever (ok maybe not that long but still) to get to the point—How do I apply this to my everyday practice?

This book is NOT a reference tome. If you were hoping it was one of the above-described mucus dripping rich texts, there's loads of those. Take this book back to where you bought and get a refund. The purpose of this book is NOT to tell you all the background knowledge on a subject, nor the basic science, nor the meaning of life.

This book is a very practical, efficient reference guide, a "get your hands dirty" kind of book. It will not put you to sleep (if it does, I will cry or work you up for a sleep disorder or both). It will give you the "gist" of the basic science, the "what do I really need to know" on each subject, and shocking information i.e., how to actually perform the procedure! This book is not for the faint of heart, nor those without a sense of humor. But, should you find yourself inclined toward the practice of allergy, you will find that the diagnosis, management, and treatment of allergy patients can be extremely rewarding. Dear reader, I hope you find this book valuable in your pursuit of allergy practice.

Your humble servant
Christine B. Franzese, MD, FAAOA

Acknowledgments

I would like to thank my fantastic and wonderful staff at the ENT and Allergy Center of Missouri for all their help and support. Also, thanks to Cindy, Jane, Dani, Elaine, Brooke, Brook, Nichole, Nick, Christy, Sarah, Carie, Ashley, Courteney, Jessie, and Will. It is such a privilege to work with you all.

Christine B. Franzese, MD

Contributors

Elizabeth J. Mahoney Davis, MD
Private practice
Newburyport, Massachusetts
Clinical Assistant Professor
Department of Otolaryngology—Head and Neck Surgery
Boston University School of Medicine
Boston, Massachusetts

Steven M. Houser, MD, FACS
Professor
Department of Otolaryngology—Head and Neck Surgery
Case Western Reserve University School of Medicine
MetroHealth Medical Center
Cleveland, Ohio

Bryan Leatherman, MD
Private practice
Coastal Sinus and Allergy Center
Gulfport, Mississippi

James W. Mims, MD
Associate Professor
Department of Otolaryngology—Head and Neck Surgery
Wake Forest School of Medicine
Wake Forest University
Winston-Salem, North Carolina

Michael J. Parker, MD
Private practice
Camillus, New York
Clinical Associate Professor
Department of Otolaryngology—Head & Neck Surgery
State University of New York Upstate Medical University
Syracuse, New York

William R. Reisacher, MD
Associate Professor
Otolaryngology
Director of Allergy Services
Department of Otolaryngology—Head & Neck Surgery
Weill Cornell Medicine
Cornell University
NewYork-Presbyterian Hospital
New York, New York

Part 1

The Basics

1 Basics of Immunology

Christine B. Franzese

1.1 Introduction

Most practicing clinicians are not necessarily skilled immunologists on the latest benchtop research. Immunology is one of the subjects that has been taught to medical students and, while important, it doesn't seem applicable in day-to-day clinical practice. However, having knowledge of the basic mechanisms involved in allergic disorders is helpful in fully understanding how treatments for these diseases work and how to maximize the benefits for the patients. In this chapter a brief review of the immunology behind type I immunoglobulin E (IgE)-mediated hypersensitivity has been described in simple terms.

1.2 Hypersensitivity Reactions

There are several different types of hypersensitivity reactions. This book deals primarily with type I IgE-mediated hypersensitivity reactions, the cause of "allergies." As implied, these reactions start very quickly (hence, the "immediate" nature of them) and the primary immunoglobulin (i.e., antibody) involved is IgE.

1.3 Adaptive Immunity

The immune system can be divided into two basic parts—the innate immune system and the adaptive immune system. The innate immune system comprises a network of barrier, enzymatic and cellular defenses that protect the body from invaders by using mechanisms that do not change or alter, regardless of what pathogens are attacking the body. The adaptive immune system comprises cellular and humoral defenses (immunoglobulins, proteins, and chemical signals) that do change or alter with the nature of the invading pathogen. It also has "memory" and its responses generally become more robust with repeated exposure to the same infection.

1.4 Adaptive Immune Responses

The adaptive immune system can respond in different ways, but it can be divided into two different types of responses based on the type of T-helper (T_h) cell involved. T_h1 responses are geared toward defense against intracellular invaders, while T_h2 responses are meant to defend against extracellular pathogens and parasites. Before progressing further, let's review the different cells that play a role in allergic disorders and their treatments.

1.5 The Major Players

Antigen presenting cells (APCs): A class of cells that begin the allergic reaction. These types of cells include dendritic cells, Langerhans cells, and other cells. When APCs come into contact with some unknown pathogen, they swallow it up, chop it up into tiny pieces, and then present those tiny pieces on their surface to show to other cells, saying, "Hey! Do you know what this is? Have you seen this before?"

T-cells: A class of white blood cells. T-cells come in different varieties, and each variety has its own roles and responsibilities within the immune system. In this chapter, only certain T-cell types will be discussed. An APC usually shows its goods to some type of T-cells in the earlier stages of infection.

T helper cells: A class of T-cells and the most important cell type in the adaptive immune system. These cells help direct other cells to make antibodies, attack infected cells, or release chemical messages. They may help activate one part of the immune system and/or suppress another. These cells direct B-cells to produce different types of antibodies.

B cells: A class of white blood cells that produce Ig. While they can function as APCs, making antibodies is pretty much what they do. T-cells send signals to B-cells to produce a specific class of antibodies.

Immunoglobulins: These cells are also known as antibodies. They comprise five different varieties: IgG, IgM, IgA, IgD, and IgE. These are proteins made by B-cells that bind to a wide range of molecules and "flag" these things for the immune system. When an antibody binds to something, Igs tell the immune system, "Hey, pay attention to this! Do something with it!"

T helper type 1 cells (T_h1): A type of T_h cell responsible for defending against intracellular bacteria, viruses, and other infections. T_h1 cells send signals to B cells and direct them to produce IgG. When overactivated or not working correctly, this arm of the immune system can lead to autoimmune diseases.

T helper type 2 cells (T_h2): A type of T_h cell responsible for defending against extracellular parasites and other infections. T_h2 cells send signals to B-cells and direct them to make IgE. When overactivated or not working correctly, this arm of the immune system leads to allergic disorders and type I IgE-mediated hypersensitivity. When you think of T_h2, think "achoo."

T regulatory cells (T_{reg}): A type of T-cell that, when working correctly, keeps the other T-cells in check, especially the T_h cells. It keeps them from getting too worked up about things, saying, "Relax, take a chill pill." These cells play an important role in the development of tolerance and in immunotherapy.

Mast cells: These white blood cells live in the body's tissues. They are essentially little floating bags of histamine and other chemical mediators. They bind IgE to their surface and when triggered, release histamine and other inflammatory mediators that cause the typical wheal and flare response (itching, redness, swelling).

Basophils: These white blood cells float in the bloodstream and are similar to, but not the same as, mast cells. They too are little floating bags of histamine and other chemical mediators. They bind IgE as well and participate in allergic diseases and anaphylaxis.

Eosinophils: A class of white blood cells that could be known as the "worm killers," due to their role in fighting extracellular parasites. They are also little floating bags of preformed chemical mediators and they migrate from the blood into a variety of organs and tissues. They play a role in allergic disorders and asthma as well.

1.6 Tolerance and Immune System Bias

The development of allergic disease depends on two basic factors. The first is a breakdown in tolerance and the other is if there is a bias in the adaptive immune response. One of the most important things the immune system does is learn to identify, recognize, and discriminate between a part of you (*self*) and what belongs to the rest of the world (*non-self*), as well as what is a threat to the self—both internal and external threats. The process by which the immune system learns to differentiate between self, non-self, and threats is called *tolerance*. When tolerance works as expected, the immune system attacks both external non-self (i.e., bacteria) and internal self-threats (i.e., malignant cells) while leaving nonthreatening non-self-things (i.e., pollen) and normal self-components alone.

When tolerance breaks down, the immune system may begin to attack things, both self and non-self, which are not threats while ignoring real internal and external threats. When this happens, allergic disorders can develop if there is a T_h2 bias to the immune system. Ideally, the different immune responses work in balance (▶ Fig. 1.1). When a shift occurs that favors one type of immune response over the other, then there is a *bias* in the immune system. If this bias favors a T_h2 response, allergic diseases develop. One of the potential benefits of immunotherapy is the reduction and potential elimination of that T_h2 bias.

1.7 A Word on the Simplification of the Immune System

In this chapter a simplified version of the immunology at work in type I IgE-mediated hypersensitivity is presented. However, the immune system is certainly not as simple and straightforward as presented here and there are nuances that are not covered. As our understanding improves and research progresses, it's become apparent that the barrier function of the innate

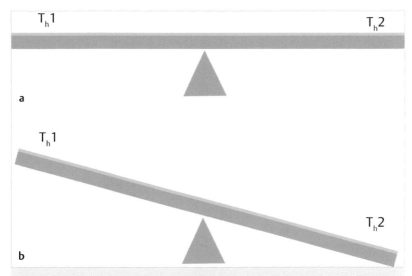

Fig. 1.1 (a) When the T_h1 and T_h2 sides of the immune system are in balance. **(b)** When the immune system has a T_h2 bias and favors a T_h2 response.

immune system isn't necessarily as simple as initially thought, and that the cells in the adaptive immune system don't always stick to their defined roles or work the way it seems they should. For example, epithelial cells not only serve as a barrier, but can also produce chemical messages that shift the immune response toward a T_h2 bias. APC too can have an innate T_h1 or T_h2 bias, depending on the circumstances. Hopefully this brief chapter serves as a straightforward refresher in immunology concepts, and encourages further exploration into this fascinating subject.

Bibliography

[1] Chaplin DD. Overview of the immune response. J Allergy Clin Immunol. 2010; 125(2) Suppl 2: S3–S23
[2] Togias AG. Systemic immunologic and inflammatory aspects of allergic rhinitis. J Allergy Clin Immunol. 2000; 106(5) Suppl:S247–S250

2 Allergic Rhinitis: Definition and Classifications

Christine B. Franzese

2.1 The Keys to Success

The best way to find a solution to a problem is to first define it. Once you know exactly what you're dealing with, you're much closer to accomplishing your goal. In immunology the goal is to determine the best type of allergy treatment for the patients. Classifying what type of allergic rhinitis patients have is useful in guiding not just the selection of what antigens you may test patients for, but also what pharmaceutical treatments you might use and determining if immunotherapy is the best option.

2.2 The Definition

What is allergic rhinitis? Allergic rhinitis is an inflammatory condition of the nasal mucosa mediated by immunoglobulin E (IgE) sensitization to an aeroallergen (type I hypersensitivity), which causes sneezing, nasal congestion, and clear nasal drainage when exposed to the allergen in question. The diagnosis of this disorder is made when a patient exhibits or gives a history of symptoms of allergic rhinitis with positive testing for IgE to one or more suspect antigens.

Local IgE production and sensitization can affect other mucosal surfaces. Thus, allergic conjunctivitis is similar in definition to allergic rhinitis, but it afflicts the eye. Allergic pharyngitis affects the pharynx, allergic laryngitis affects the larynx, and allergic asthma affects the lungs.

2.3 The Not-So-Perfect Classification System

The classification of allergic rhinitis is dependent on the timing and persistence of symptoms and how the disease has evolved over the years. Most practitioners are familiar with the terms "seasonal" and "perennial." The Allergic Rhinitis in Asthma (ARIA) guidelines introduced new terms because the older terms didn't quite seem to fully describe the different types of allergic rhinitis. The ARIA guidelines recommend that the newer terms should not be used along with the older terminology. However, it's still very common to use older words, or even combine them with the newer ones (despite what the guidelines say), as the ARIA guideline terms also don't cover all the types either.

It is important to use the chosen terms or classification system routinely and remain consistent (not just in your own practice, but with any partners you have, as well). Documenting the timing of symptoms is key to selecting antigens for testing and treatment. Classifying the type of allergic rhinitis helps solidify that timing in your documentation. Some classification terms are discussed further, the "*" denotes terminology from the ARIA guidelines.

Seasonal: Symptoms occur during one or more seasons of the year. Generally caused by one or more outdoor allergens, typically pollens.

> Different pollens peak during different seasons; so, it's important to note during which season(s) or months of the year the symptoms occur.

Intermittent*: Symptoms occur for less than 4 days per week or less than 4 consecutive weeks. This doesn't equate to seasonal allergic rhinitis, although the tendency is to think of these terms that way.

> Still document what month(s) or time(s) of the year symptoms occur.

Exposure-related: Symptoms occur when exposed to a particular allergen, e.g., patients develop symptoms when around a cat or other animal.

> Note the specific exposure and symptoms. For example, hamsters cause some patients to have allergic conjunctivitis.

Perennial: Symptoms occur year-round or at any time of the year; generally caused by indoor allergens such as cockroaches, molds, and dust mites.

> Exposure-related allergens can cause perennial (or persistent) symptoms, as in the cat-allergic patient who owns one or more cats.

Persistent*: Symptoms occur for more than 4 days per week or at least 4 consecutive weeks or most of the time. Again, this term isn't supposed to equate perennial even though it seems like it should.

Being as specific as possible with the timing of symptom increases your accuracy in selecting culprit antigens. I personally mix these terms to capture the most accurate picture (i.e., "perennial rhinitis with spring/fall seasonal flareups," "cat-exposure perennial rhinitis,") as it's pretty common for patients to present with a mixed picture.

2.4 Severity

Quality-of-life questionnaires can be helpful in capturing severity of symptoms, but if you don't use them, be sure to rate or note the severity of patient symptoms. This is helpful in discussing treatment options with a patient. When considering immunotherapy, the greater the severity of symptoms a patient has, the more likely that patient will perceive improvement from immunotherapy, and the more likely he/she will be compliant. A patient with mild short-lived symptoms in one season who responds well to a single medication doesn't need immunotherapy, and arguably is not a good candidate for it. While technically immunotherapy will likely "make him/her better," the question is whether it will make them "better enough" to really notice it and be compliant with therapy.

Clinical Pearls   M!

- Classification is based on timing of symptoms.
- Be as specific as possible for timing/exposures.
- Pay attention to severity of symptoms when considering/discussing treatment options.

Bibliography

[1] Bousquet J, Van Cauwenberge P, Khaltaev N, Aria Workshop Group, World Health Organization. Allergic rhinitis and its impact on asthma. J Allergy Clin Immunol. 2001; 108(5) Suppl:S147–S334

[2] Wallace DV, Dykewicz MS, Bernstein DI, et al. Joint Task Force on Practice, American Academy of Allergy, Asthma & Immunology, American College of Allergy, Asthma and Immunology, Joint Council of Allergy, Asthma and Immunology. The diagnosis and management of rhinitis: an updated practice parameter. J Allergy Clin Immunol. 2008; 122(2) Suppl:S1–S84

3 Sensitization versus Allergy

Christine B. Franzese

3.1 A Most Interesting Conundrum

"I'm allergic to (*insert noun here—life, the State of Missouri, etc*)." Anyone who practices allergy for even a short period of time will come across some difficult situations that can cause practitioner and/or patient frustration. One of these scenarios is the patient with numerous positive allergy tests, regardless of whether it is skin or blood testing. Oddly, patients in this scenario tend to react in one of two main ways—the first reaction being an acceptance that they are truly "allergic" to everything, consigned to atopic doom, and that you must absolutely treat them with everything for which they have positive tests. But, are they truly "allergic" to everything?

The second way a patient found to have numerous positives can react, "Your tests must be wrong, Doc/I don't understand—I've been exposed to (*insert noun here—cats, dust, the summer season, etc.*) and don't have any problems." Without proper explanation, this can lead to patient confusion, misunderstanding (a false acceptance of allergy when there is none), or mistrust of the testing process or the practitioner (*"I'm not allergic to my dog, this quack has no idea how to do this"*). Without proper understanding on the practitioner's part, this can lead to overtreatment, unnecessary avoidance, and lack of perceived treatment benefit.

3.2 Serious Stuff

What is sensitization? In this case, sensitization is the demonstration of immunoglobulin E (IgE) antibodies to one or more antigens. The type of testing (skin vs. blood) is irrelevant, because if the patient is sensitized, there will be one or more positive allergy tests. The key here is that sensitization does not equal symptoms. It is important to understand that sensitization is not same as having clinical symptoms.

What is allergy? In this case, allergy is the correlation of clinical symptoms (i.e., sneezing, itching, etc.) with exposure to an antigen *plus* a positive allergy test result (skin or blood), indicating the presence of IgE antibodies to that particular antigen. For example, a patient with a positive skin test result to cat has nasal congestion when exposed to cats. This is allergy.

So you're saying my patient who had positive test results (skin or blood) for dust mites but has no symptoms on exposure to dust isn't allergic to dust mites? Technically, yes. This is an example of sensitization without clinical allergy. While the patient demonstrates IgE to dust mites, there's no correlation to clinical symptoms.

But, the test results were super positive! Huge wheals on skin testing (or massive levels of IgE)! They MUST be allergic! No. This is one of the frustrating things about allergy. The actual level of sensitization does not necessarily correlate with the severity or presence of allergy symptoms. A patient with barely positive allergy test results may have serious or life-threatening reactions on exposure; on the contrary, a patient with markedly positive test results may have very mild, barely troublesome symptoms. The presence of a positive test result by itself indicates sensitization, not allergy.

Why does this happen? Well, we're not completely sure. Some of this is due to the cross-reactivity of different antigens and the sharing of epitopes at a molecular level. There are some recent data suggesting that it's not just the presence of IgE that is important, but the ratio of IgE to IgG (or more specifically IgG4) that may help distinguish patients with sensitization only from those with clinical allergy. However, there's not enough evidence at this point to recommend ordering antigen-specific IgG4 routinely.

What if the patient forgot she/he has symptoms? This happens. Allergy patients are notorious for thinking their symptoms are "normal." There are a number of patients who have told the author with a straight face that "normal people can't breathe out of their nose." Particularly for patients with year-round allergies, these symptoms tend to become their "normal" and they may not report them to you or view them as significant. It's something they've lived with for so long, it's just become the way things are for them. However, after testing, once attention has been drawn to certain antigens, patients will sometimes put two and two together and figure out after the fact that they really do have problems with that particular antigen.

So, if the patient wants immunotherapy, what do I treat for? Allergy is a history of symptoms on exposure *with* a positive test result, so only treat for antigens that meet this definition. It is not recommended that the patient should be treated for antigens that only demonstrate sensitization.

> ⚠️
>
> Have a place on your skin testing form for your testing personnel to check boxes or list what symptoms the patient has, timing/seasonality of symptoms, and exposures (pets, etc.). This makes it easier to discuss results with the patient and select antigens for treatment, without have to go back into your notes to find this information.

So, what do I do now? How you handle each patient depends upon the situation, but generally comes down to patient education and counseling. Easier said than done. Positive test results without symptoms can cause quite a bit of mischief for you and your patient.

3.3 Mischief Management

Scenario one: *The patient is "allergic to life."* While it's quite possible the patient is truly allergic to everything he/she tested positive for, it's also likely they're not. Certainly, the risk of allergic disease increases with the quantity of sensitizations, but you also have to keep in mind cross-reactivity and the presence of symptoms. The best you can do in this scenario is to match symptoms on exposure to positive test results. If the patient professes to have symptoms year-round with peaks in every season and on all exposures, then you have to use your best clinical judgment as to what antigens are most relevant to the patient and treat for those.

It is not recommended to convince a patient in this scenario that they are "not allergic" to something. More often than not, trying to do so will not go well at all. Rather, discuss with the patient what they *are* (which is sensitized), rather than what they *are not*.

Scenario two: *Your tests are wrong.* While no test is perfect, allergy testing via skin and/or blood is pretty reliable. While you can discuss the false-positive rates of skin or blood testing, patients in this scenario are much more receptive to a discussion of sensitization versus allergy. This discussion tends to be a lot better with the patient than a discussion of the flaws of the method you used to test them for allergies. These patients also tend to be more receptive to explanations regarding the cross-reactivity of certain antigens.

3.4 One Last Frustration...

"Your tests must be wrong, Doc/I don't understand—I AM allergic to (insert noun here—cats, dust, the summer season, etc.) and have symptoms when exposed."

This is the dreaded scenario when a patient who comes in for allergy testing and has negative test results to everything, including things to which he/she may have symptoms. While uncommon, it happens so be prepared for it. No tests are perfect and you should be knowledgeable about different testing methods if this happens. It is reasonable to discuss, using a different method of testing, with patients who have given a history that strongly suggests allergy. However, not every symptom is IgE-mediated and not all things can be blamed on allergic disease. Be prepared to discuss and treat other disorders in your differential, such as irritant rhinitis. If allergy medications, such as antihistamines or nasal steroid sprays, work for the patient, continue them. Under no circumstances should you initiate immunotherapy for an antigen which has negative test results. Immunotherapy treats IgE-mediated allergic disease and until you have evidence that a particularly antigen had IgE to it, immunotherapy is not indicated for that antigen.

Clinical Pearls   **M!**

- Sensitization is positive allergy test results (skin or blood).
- Allergy is sensitization *plus* a history of corresponding symptoms.
- Do not treat allergens that do not have positive test results.
- Match symptoms to test results to help guide what antigens to treat.

Bibliography

[1] Carroll WD, Lenney W, Child F, et al. Asthma severity and atopy: how clear is the relationship? Arch Dis Child. 2006; 91(5):405–409

[2] Johansson SG, Bieber T, Dahl R, et al. Revised nomenclature for allergy for global use: Report of the Nomenclature Review Committee of the World Allergy Organization, October 2003. J Allergy Clin Immunol. 2004; 113(5):832–836

[3] Roberts G, Ollert M, Aalberse R, et al. A new framework for the interpretation of IgE sensitization tests. Allergy. 2016; 71(11):1540–1551

4 Unified Airway Concept

Christine B. Franzese

4.1 What It Is

There are different classifications of rhinitis or "phenotypes," such as allergic rhinitis, nonallergic rhinitis, and mixed rhinitis. There are also different types of asthma, such as allergic, nonallergic, and mixed phenotypes. These different classifications or types of rhinitis and asthma seem very similar or overlap. This similarity is vital in understanding the unified airway concept: the idea that the upper and lower respiratory tracts are linked, not just anatomically, but also through pathophysiology and mechanisms of inflammation; that inflammation in the upper respiratory tract can influence the lower respiratory tract (and vice versa) as part of a single system. This concept also helps emphasize that type I-mediated hypersensitivity is a systemic phenomenon and that allergic inflammation isn't necessarily isolated to one area.

4.2 How Might This Work?

This concept is based on the foundation that allergic inflammation is a systemic process and that inflammatory signals and cells travel through the bloodstream from one site to another. This is best modeled in studies where an allergen is introduced into either the nasal airway (nasal challenge) or lungs (bronchial challenge), but not both at the same time. Generally, it is seen that exposing one part of the respiratory system (either upper or lower) leads to allergic inflammation in both parts.

4.3 What About Postnasal Drip? Can That Cause Lung Inflammation?

It was assumed that inflammatory mediators present in "postnasal drip" (thickened nasal mucus that flows down the pharynx) may influence inflammation in the lungs. However, there's no solid evidence to support this and in an anatomic and physiologic sense, this idea doesn't work. Unless one has a true vocal cord paralysis, laryngeal tumor, or some other disease that alters the function and/or structure of your larynx, there is no direct contact between upper airway tract and the lower respiratory tract. In fact, the larynx has protective reflexes to help prevent aspiration of secretions. While nasal mucus does flow down the pharynx, it's generally swallowed and not aspirated. A study has found deposits of radioactively labeled allergens applied to the nasal airway in the gastrointestinal tract and not in the lungs.

4.4 Why It Is Important

In the clinical treatment of patients, it is important to understand how the upper and lower airways influence each other. Reducing inflammation or hyperreactivity in one part of the airway may improve the clinical symptoms in the other part. In addition, newer medications, surgical procedures, and/or biologic agents that target inflammatory mediators may affect one or both areas so this understanding may help the clinician in the selection of what treatment options to use. However, this concept isn't perfect and there are no guarantees that improving symptoms in one area will help improve symptoms in the other. For example, in some asthmatic patients, chronic sinusitis can worsen their asthma and endoscopic surgical procedures that reduce sinus inflammation seem to improve those patients' lung function; however, in other asthmatics, improving sinus inflammation may have no impact on their asthma status. The clinician should keep in mind that with regards to allergic inflammation, it's all one airway.

Clinical Pearls **M!**

- Systemic inflammatory mediators can affect both the upper and lower respiratory tracts.
- Be sure to screen for potential asthma for allergic rhinitis patients.
- Be sure to weigh the potential impact of sinusitis and allergic rhinitis on lower respiratory function for asthmatic patients.

Bibliography

[1] Bagnasco M, Mariani G, Passalacqua G, et al. Absorption and distribution kinetics of the major Parietaria judaica allergen (Par j 1) administered by noninjectable routes in healthy human beings. J Allergy Clin Immunol. 1997; 100(1):122–129

[2] Braunstahl GJ. United airways concept: what does it teach us about systemic inflammation in airways disease? Proc Am Thorac Soc. 2009; 6(8):652–654

[3] Genuneit J, Seibold AM, Apfelbacher CJ, et al. Task Force 'Overview of Systematic Reviews in Allergy Epidemiology (OSRAE)' of the EAACI Interest Group on Epidemiology. Overview of systematic reviews in allergy epidemiology. Allergy. 2017; 72(6):849–856

5 Inhalant Allergens: Grasses

Steven M. Houser, Sarah K. Wise

5.1 When Summer Isn't Something to Look Forward To

Grass pollen can be a potent allergen for sensitized individuals and is typically present during the summer months, especially early summer. There are three subfamilies of grasses that are most common in the United States: Pooideae, Cloridodeae, and Panicoideae. Cross-reactivity among grasses is high within subfamilies. It is important to understand allergen cross-reactivity and standardization in order to provide excellent care for the allergy patient.

5.2 Serious Stuff

5.2.1 Quick Review... What Is an Antigen? And What Is an Allergen?

An *antigen* is a substance, most commonly a protein or polysaccharide, that causes the body to produce an antibody. The part of the antigen that is recognized by the body's immune system is the *epitope*. The *paratope* is the part of the antibody that recognizes the antigen epitope. The epitope-paratope configuration that occurs upon antigen-antibody recognition is a unique three-dimensional lock-and-key formation. Of note, some epitopes from different antigens may be sufficiently similar in structure to bind the same antibody paratope; this results in *cross-reactivity*. An *allergen* is antigen that specifically triggers the allergic cascade; an allergen epitope binds paratopes on immunoglobulin E (IgE) molecules.

5.2.2 Tell Me a Bit More About Allergens... Please?

Substances containing allergenic proteins and polysaccharides are frequently complex biological constructs (e.g., pollen spores), and they often contain multiple proteins with varied epitopes. Certain allergens are identified as more important than the others. A *major allergen* is an antigenic fraction to which at least 50% of patients are sensitive per in vitro or in vivo testing. A minor allergen causes less than 50% of patients to react. For example, the major allergen in cat dander extract is Fel d 1, but the extract can contain multiple minor allergens as well. Understandably, patients will vary in their reactivity to major and minor allergens. Multiple major allergens have been identified and are noted throughout this and other inhalant allergen chapters.

A vial of allergen extract contains multiple components including the major and minor allergens themselves, as well as inert proteins and extract solution. Most nonstandardized extracts are preserved in a 50% glycerin solution ± 0.4% phenol. Extracts will deteriorate over time with a typical shelf life of ≤ 3 years at 4 °C.

5.2.3 What Are Standardized and Nonstandardized Allergen Extracts?

For the most part, allergy extracts have been only roughly quantified, although more strict standardization is evolving. Nonstandardized quantification schemes include allergen units (Noon units, 1 unit of pollen toxin from 1,000th part of 1 mg Phleum pollen), protein nitrogen units (PNU, 0.01 µg of phospho-tungstic acid-precipitable protein nitrogen), and weight per volume (W/V). The last method is the most commonly used method: the weight (grams) of dry allergen in a volume (100 mL) of solution. Bioequivalence will be roughly maintained within a company through consistent manufacturing, but significant variation will exist between manufacturers.

Standardized extracts date back to 1981 and are extracts which have been tested to be equivalent to a recognized reference. The Food and Drug Administration (FDA) produces a reference standard and manufacturers compare their product lot with this standard. If a sample's activity is between 70% and 140% of the reference standard then the lot passes and is designated the same bioequivalent allergy unit (BAU) concentration as the standard. Multiple standardization methods exist. Grass allergens are standardized via radioallergosorbent (RAST) or enzyme-linked immunosorbent assay (ELISA) inhibition. Standards for dust mite are referenced using three fold dilutions, similar to the five-fold dilutions used for intradermal dilutional testing, although erythema size, not wheal, is measured. Cat is standardized by assaying major allergen content (Fel d 1). If a standardized allergen exists, then it is best to use the standardized allergen instead of its W/V quantified option; the bioactivity across lots and manufacturers is more consistent and hence safer. Standardized extracts are quantified in allergy units (AU) for dust mites, BAUs for some allergens (e.g., cat, grasses), or major allergen content in micrograms (e.g., short ragweed Amb a1). Some of the current standardized allergens licensed within the United States are discussed throughout this and other inhalant allergen chapters.

5.2.4 What Is Cross-Reactivity?

Cross-reactivity is a concept that must be understood to fully appreciate the complexities of allergy management. As many plants share a common evolutionary history, their allergens (and epitopes) will be conserved or minimally changed between species. Cross-reactivity increases with the closeness of the biologic relationship: order → family → (tribe within a family) → genus →

species (the latter are most closely related). Cross-reactivity between intimately related species is common. Hence the body may react to two different pollinating species of plant interchangeably as the "lock and key" of antigen to IgE (epitope to paratope) molecule is similar. When an individual reacts similarly to different species, these species are described as being cross-reactive. In general, grasses tend to have the most cross-reactivity, weeds to a lesser degree, and trees possess the least cross-reactivity. Cross-reactivity can also occur between unrelated inhalants, and between foods and inhalants, if they happen to contain similar epitopes. An example is orally ingested apples and inhaled birch pollen that contain similar epitopes; a birch-sensitive patient can develop oral itching/swelling (oral allergy syndrome) from eating apples.

5.2.5 What Are Thommen's Postulates?

Plant-derived allergens differ geographically, depending upon the prevalent species in a particular area and the local climate (▶ Fig. 5.1). In 1931, Thommen's postulates were proposed. These are helpful to explain what constitutes an allergenic plant. These rules include:
1. The pollen must be wind-borne, or *anemophilus*. Insect-pollinated plants are termed *entomophilus*. Pollens from entomophilus plants tend to be heavy and sticky; these pollens do not trigger allergic responses unless present in overwhelming concentrations. *Amphiphilous* plants combine the two strategies discussed and use both wind and insects for pollination.
2. The pollen must be produced in large quantities.
3. The pollen must be light enough to travel a long distance on the wind currents.
4. The plant must be broadly distributed within the environment.
5. The pollen must contain allergens capable of causing an allergic response.

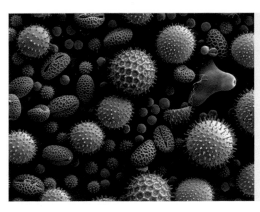

Fig. 5.1 Pollen grains seen under scanning electron microscopy.

5.2.6 What Exactly Is Pollen?

A pollen particle is the male germinal cell (gametophyte) used for plant reproduction. Most aeroallergen pollen grains are 15 to 50 µm in diameter (▶ Fig. 5.1). The germinal center is surrounded by a vaguely spherical rigid wall of polysaccharide material termed *sporopollenin*. Pollen grains are produced in the microsporangium of the plant and released passively into the environment to reach the receptive female stigma. A pollen allergen is typically a low-molecular-weight molecule (5–60 kDa) carried on a pollen particle that diffuses rapidly into an aqueous solution upon contact. For example, when a pollen grain strikes the nasal membrane, allergens diffuse away from the firm structure to be encountered by IgE molecules on the surface of mast cells. Pollen and/or its allergenic particles may also be aerosolized in smaller fragments allowing the material to bypass nasal filtering and reach the lungs. Pollens are typically released during the morning, and patients may experience aggravation of symptoms at that time. Dry, windy days will elevate pollen counts while damp, rainy weather will temporarily reduce the counts.

5.2.7 What Types of Plants Produce Allergenic Pollens?

The two major categories of pollen-producing plants are *gymnosperms* and *angiosperms*. Gymnosperms carry their ovules "naked" on the scales of a cone or on the end of short stalks. Examples of gymnosperms include nonflowering trees (e.g., ginkgo) and conifers. The majority of pollen-producing plants are angiosperms; their sex organs are within flowers and their seeds are usually located within a fruit. The term angiosperm encompasses flowering trees, grasses, and weeds. The United States is divided into 11 zones based upon the climate and flora in these regions. As pollens are geography-specific, it is imperative that one identifies the species in their area to guide allergy testing and treatment.

5.2.8 What Are Some Highlights About Grass Allergens?

Grass pollens are among the most potent allergens produced in nature and have been reported to be the most prevalent cause of allergic rhinitis worldwide. However, of approximately 4,500 grass species worldwide, only a small number are of allergenic importance. Up to 50 antigens have been identified in grass pollens, including 10 allergen groups. Grass pollen antigens include plant proteins such as expansins and calcium-binding proteins. Grasses are strongly cross-reactive within their subfamilies, and with some foods.

The common grasses can be divided into five subfamilies. Three of these subfamilies are most important in North America: Pooideae, Cloridodeae, and Panicoideae. The remaining two subfamilies may also have local importance: Arundinoideae and Bambusoideae.

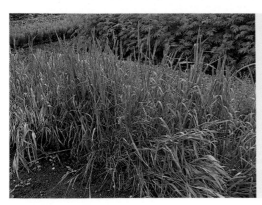

Fig. 5.2 Timothy grass.

The Pooideae subfamily contains most of the cultivated and wild grasses throughout the world, including brome, fescue, June, Orchard, perennial rye, redtop, sweet vernal, timothy, and Kentucky blue grasses. Most cereal grains are of this subfamily, including barley, oats, rye, spelt, and wheat. Epitopes are widely shared within this subfamily, resulting in strong cross-reactivity. Timothy pollen appears to contain all of these important epitopes (i.e., Phl p 1, 4, 5) (▶ Fig. 5.2).

The Cloridodeae subfamily is most important on the central plains and subtropics but does have representation in most regions of North America. Bermuda, Buffalo, Grama, and Zoysia grasses are prominent members of this group. The members of this group display strong cross-reactivity within their subfamily, and minor cross-reactivity with other grasses. Bermuda grass pollen contains most of the epitopes produced by this subfamily (i.e., Cyn d 1).

The Panicoideae subfamily is common in the southern part of North America; it includes bahia, barnyard, Johnson, and crabgrasses. Edible members of this subfamily include corn (maize), millet, sorghum (molasses), and sugarcane. This subfamily displays limited cross-reactivity with other grasses. Bahia grass appears to be the most antigenically unique of the subfamily; bahia and Johnson grass are considered the most important in the subfamily.

Timothy grass, perennial rye, Orchard, Kentucky blue (June), redtop, meadow fescue, sweet vernal, and Bermuda grasses are standardized grass allergens licensed in the United States. All of these allergens except Bermuda grass come from the Pooideae subfamily.

5.2.9 When Do Grasses Pollinate?

Plants bloom during a specific period of the year. This blooming period is linked to the local climate and intimately related to temperature, wind, moisture, etc. When plants bloom, their pollens are released. Plants that release pollen into the air (and meet Thommen's postulates) are capable of triggering an allergic individual's sensitivities, and thus, their clinical symptoms. A specific geographical location possesses some consistency in climactic factors, allowing predictions of the initiation and length of pollination. In general, grasses pollinate in the summer in the United States. Warmer climates tend to permit a lengthier growing season and pollen production, and grasses in milder climates can pollinate nearly year-round.

5.2.10 What Are Some Common Allergenic Grasses?

The following box (Box 5.1) lists some of the most common allergenic grasses:

Grasses (angiosperm): Poaceae family
Pooideae subfamily
Timothy, brome, bluegrass, redtop, June grass, Orchard, fescue, sweet vernal, barley, oat, wheat, spelt, rye
Panicoideae subfamily
Bahia, Johnson, St. Augustine, crabgrass, barnyard, corn, sugarcane, millet, sorghum (molasses)
Chloridoideae subfamily
Bermuda, Buffalo, Zoysia, Grama
Bambusoideae subfamily
Bamboo, rice
Arundinoideae subfamily
Reed

Clinical Pearls   M!

- Pollen allergens are an important source of sensitivity for the allergic patient, especially grasses.
- Grasses typically pollinate in the early summer, with specific pollination periods that vary depending on geography and climate.
- Some grasses are available as standardized allergen extracts.
- Certain grass subfamilies demonstrate substantial cross-reactivity among the grasses within them.

Bibliography

[1] Burge HA, Rogers CA. Outdoor allergens. Environ Health Perspect. 2000; 108 Suppl 4:653–659

[2] Cox L, Nelson H, Lockey R, et al. Allergen immunotherapy: a practice parameter third update. J Allergy Clin Immunol. 2011; 127(1) Suppl:S1–S55

[3] Joint Task Force on Practice Parameters. Allergen Immunotherapy. Ann Allergy Asthma Immunol. 2003; 90(1) Suppl 1:1–40

[4] Kaplan AP, ed. Allergy. Philadelphia, PA: W.B. Saunders Company; 1997

[5] King HC, Mabry RL, Mabry CS, et al, eds. Allergy in ENT Practice: The Basic Guide. New York, NY: Thieme; 2005

[6] Krouse JH, Chadwick SJ, Gordon BR, Derebery MJ, eds. Allergy and Immunology: An Otolayngic Approach. New York, NY: Lippincott Williams & Wilkins; 2002

[7] Nolte H. Optimal maintenance dose immunotherapy based on major allergen content or potency labeling. Allergy. 1998; 53(1):99–100

[8] Patterson R, Grammer LC, Greenberger PA, eds. Allergic Diseases: Diagnosis and Management. New York, NY: Lippincott Williams & Wilkins; 1997

[9] Krouse JH, Chadwick SJ, Parker MJ. Inhalant allergy. In: Krouse JH, Chadwick SJ, Gordon BR, Derebery MJ, eds. Allergy and Immunology: An Otolaryngic Approach. Philadelphia, PA: Lippincott-Williams & Wilkins; 2002: 35-49

6 Inhalant Allergens: Trees

Steven M. Houser, Sarah K. Wise

6.1 Springtime Tree Troubles

Tree pollen is prevalent in the springtime, and patients with spring allergy symptoms are often reacting to tree pollen. With the exception of the cypress family, gymnosperm trees tend to have pollen that is milder in antigenicity. Angiosperms are diverse and more antigenic. It is important to understand the cross-reactivity among trees, as this may occur at the genus or family level. Some major allergens have been identified for trees, although there are no standardized allergen extracts available for trees commercially in the United States at this time.

Please see Chapter 5 for a review of the following topics:
- Definition of antigen, allergen, epitope.
- Major versus minor allergens.
- Allergen extract units, standardized versus non-standardized allergen extracts.
- Cross-reactivity.
- Thommen's postulates.
- Description of pollen particles and the plants that produce pollen.

6.2 Serious Stuff

6.2.1 What Are the Common Types of Allergenic Trees in North America?

The symptoms of spring allergy are often attributed to the pollination of trees. Trees have the greatest diversity among plants and are the least cross-reactive. Trees tend to cross-react strongly at the genus level, but typically not at the broader family level.

Gymnosperm trees produce copious pollen, but tend to be milder in allergenicity. For example, conifers produce buoyant pollen capable of traveling hundreds of miles and coating cars, windows, etc., yet it is less allergenic. A notable exception is the cypress family (Cupressaceae), including mountain cedar, which can have very potent pollens. The mountain cedar, *Juniperus ashei* (alternatively *Juniperus sabinoides* or *Juniperus mexicana*) is the most allergenic tree in Central Texas (▶ Fig. 6.1). It is an evergreen tree with grey-brown shredding bark growing to a maximum height of approximately 30 feet and pollinating from November through March. *Cryptomeria japonica* (sugi) is another potent gymnosperm being the most prevalent tree pollen source in Japan. The

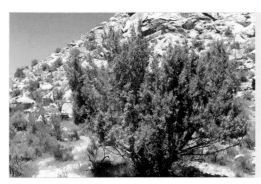

Fig. 6.1 Mountain cedar tree.

pine family (Pinaceae) produces impotent pollen, but can be an important allergen if located sufficiently close to human habitats. In addition to pines, Pinaceae includes spruce, hemlock, and fir trees. Though common, ginkgos and yew trees are not potent allergen producers. While gymnosperm families share little cross-reactivity in general, cypress family members do share major cross-reactivity.

Angiosperm trees are quite diverse and prolific. Because of their diversity, cross-reactivity commonly occurs at a genus level. In violation of this genus-only cross-reactivity rule though, some notable familial cross-reactors include: (1) birch, alder, and hazelnut; (2) oak and beech; (3) various maples with one another; and (4) olive, ash, lilac, and privet are also capable of cross-reacting. Australian pines are an angiosperm tree, not a gymnosperm pine. Poplars and cotton woods produce seeds with cottony tufts and release them during summer season. These are often falsely blamed for allergy symptoms during summer, while tree pollen production occurs early in the year. Despite the fact that trees are geographic-specific, in general, oak (▶ Fig. 6.2) is considered the most important allergenic tree in North America, while birch carries the same distinction in Europe. Due to the limited cross-reactivity among this group, the members should be tested for and treated individually specific for the practice location.

6.2.2 When Do Trees Pollinate?

The typical season for tree pollination in North America is the springtime. Allergy patients with symptoms during this time may be reacting to tree pollen aeroallergens.

6.2.3 What Are Some Common Allergenic Trees?

The box (Box 6.1) lists some common allergenic trees.

Trees

<u>Gymnosperm</u>

Pinaceae family
  Pine, spruce, hemlock, fir
Ginkoaceae family
  Ginkgo
Tacaceae family
  Yew
Taxodiceae family
  Redwood, bald cypress
Cupressaceae family
  Juniper, mountain cedar, sugi, cypress, arborvitae

<u>Angiosperm</u>

Aceraceae family
  Maple, box elder
Anacardiaceae family
  Cashew, mango, poison ivy
Betulaceae family
  Birch, alder, hazelnut
Casuarinaceae family
  Australian pine
Fagaceae family
  Oak, beech
Juglandaceae family
  Walnut, hickory, pecan
Oleaceae family
  Olive, ash, lilac, privet
Platanaceae family
  Sycamore
Salicaceae family
  Aspen, cottonwood, poplar, willow
Ulmaceae family
  Elm
Arecaceae family
  Palm, palmetto, date palm

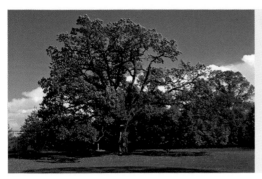

Fig. 6.2 Oak tree.

6.2.4 Which Trees Have Major Allergens That Are Known?

The following trees have had major allergens identified:
- Olive tree pollen: Ole e I.
- European birch: Bet v1, 2.
- European alder: Aln g 1.
- Sugi: Cry j 1.

6.2.5 Which Trees Have Standard Allergen Extracts Available?

Tree extracts are not available in standardized form in the United States at this time.

Clinical Pearls　　　　　　　　　　　　　　　**M!**

- Trees are an important source of springtime pollen and allergy symptoms.
- Gymnosperms tend to be less allergenic with the notable exception of the cypress family.
- Angiosperms are diverse and more allergenic.
- The medical provider should have a proper understanding of cross-reactivity among trees in order to provide the best care for the allergy patient.

Bibliography

[1] Kaplan AP, ed. Allergy. Philadelphia, PA: W.B. Saunders Company; 1997
[2] Wahl R, Schmid-Grendelmeier P, Cromwell O, Wüthrich B. In vitro investigation of cross-reactivity between birch and ash pollen allergen extracts. J Allergy Clin Immunol. 1996; 98(1):99–106

7 Inhalant Allergens: Molds

Steven M. Houser, Sarah K. Wise

7.1 Spores Can Get You Down

Mold allergy can affect patients year-round or seasonally, depending on the environment. Molds are diverse, with over 1 million species reported. From an allergy standpoint, molds may be involved in type I immunoglobulin E (IgE)-mediated reactions or type IV cell-mediated reactions. Several different molds commonly cause IgE-mediated reactivity and are often seen on allergy testing panels.

Please see Chapter 5 for a review of the following topics:
- Definition of antigen, allergen, epitope.
- Major versus minor allergens.
- Allergen extract units, standardized versus nonstandardized allergen extracts.
- Cross-reactivity.

7.2 Serious Stuff

7.2.1 What Do I Need to Know About Mold Allergy?

The term *fungus* is often used interchangeably with mold. The organisms in this kingdom were classified by their micro- and macroscopic appearance in the past, which was cumbersome given different stages/appearances during their life cycle. Nowadays genomic analysis is being used frequently to place fungi into taxonomic groupings. Kingdom Fungi can be divided into 1 subkingdom (Dikarya), 7 phyla, and 10 subphyla.

Ascomycota is a phylum within the subkingdom Dikarya; this group is often referred to as Sac fungi. Sac fungi are useful for making bread, cheese, and alcohol (baker's and brewer's yeast) and antibiotics (*Penicillium*). Three subphyla within Ascomycota include Saccharomycotina (yeasts and Candida), Taphrinomycotina (hyphal fungi and *Pneumocystis*), and Pezizomycotina (truffles and *Trichophyton*). *Cladosporium, Penicillium, Fusarium, Curvularia, Helminthosporium, Bipolaris, Phoma, Epicoccum,* and *Aspergillus* are members of Pezizomycotina family and recognized as allergenic in humans, and are often pathogenic to plants.

The Basidiomycota phylum, also within Dikarya, includes complex structural fungi such as mushrooms, puffballs, smuts, and rusts. It also includes the pathogenic yeast *Cryptococcus.*

The phylum Glomeromycota typically forms a symbiotic relationship with plant roots. Important genera include *Mucor, Rhizomucor,* and *Rhizopus.* The remaining six fungal phyla include Microsporidia, Blastocladiomycota, Zoopagomycotina, Kichxellomycotina, Entomophthoromycotina, and Mucoro-mycotina.

Clinicians should be aware that mold extracts, as well as cockroach, contain proteolytic enzymes that may degrade pollen antigens; therefore these agents should not be instilled into a common treatment vial. Cross-reactivity of molds is very complex and unpredictable, although it is known that *Alternaria* and *Cladosporium* cross-react. General recommendations for allergy skin testing panels tend to include *Alternaria, Aspergillus, Cladosporium, Helminthosporium,* and *Penicillium.*

7.2.2 What Are Some Common Allergenic Molds?

The box below (Box 7.1) demonstrates the kingdom Fungi. Common allergenic molds are highlighted in bold.

Fungi kingdom
  Dikarya subkingdom
    Ascomycota phylum
      Saccharomycotina: Yeasts and **Candida**
      Taphrinomycotina: Hyphal fungi and Pneumocystis
      Pezizomycotina: Truffles, Trichophyton, and many allergenic molds:
        Cladosporium, Penicillium, Fusarium, Curvularia, Helminthosporium, Bipolaris, Phoma, Epicoccum, and **Aspergillus**
      Basidiomycota phylum: Mushrooms, puffballs, smuts and rusts, Cryptococcus

  Glomeromycota phylum: **Mucor** and **Rhizopus**

7.2.3 Which Molds Have Major Allergens That Are Known?

The following molds have had major allergens identified:
- *Aspergillus fumigatus*: Ag 7; Ag 13 (antigen C).
- *Alternaria alternata*: One major antigen (Ag 8), seven intermediate, and six minor allergens.
- *Candida albicans*: C and a.

7.2.4 Which Molds Have Standard Allergen Extracts Available?

Mold extracts are not available commercially in standardized form in the United States at this time.

Clinical Pearls	**M!**

- Molds may cause allergic sensitivity and clinical allergy manifestations.
- Cross-reactivity among molds is complex and can be unpredictable.
- The most commonly tested molds on allergy panels are *Alternaria* and *Aspergillus*; however, *Cladosporium, Helminthosporium,* and *Penicillium* are also often recommended.

Bibliography

[1] Cox L, Nelson H, Lockey R, et al. Allergen immunotherapy: a practice parameter third update. J Allergy Clin Immunol. 2011; 127(1) Suppl:S1–S55

[2] Hibbett DS, Binder M, Bischoff JF, et al. A higher-level phylogenetic classification of the Fungi. Mycol Res. 2007; 111(Pt 5):509–547

[3] Lutzoni F, Kauff F, Cox CJ, et al. Assembling the fungal tree of life: progress, classification, and evolution of subcellular traits. Am J Bot. 2004; 91(10):1446–1480

8 Inhalant Allergens: Epidermals and Danders

Steven M. Houser, Sarah K. Wise

8.1 Dust and Danders

Dust mites and animal proteins are an important source of allergenic material that is typically present year-round. Some patients are highly reactive to these substances. The most common dust mites are *Dermatophagoides farinae* (North America) and *D. pteronyssinus* (Europe). Cat and dog allergens may be a substantial source of allergic symptoms for pet owners and other exposed individuals.

Please see Chapter 5 for a review of the following topics:
- Definition of antigen, allergen, and epitope.
- Major versus minor allergens.
- Allergen extract units, standardized versus nonstandardized allergen extracts.
- Cross-reactivity.

8.2 Serious Stuff

8.2.1 What Potential Allergens Do We Encounter Year-Round?

A variety of fauna are potential sources of clinically significant aeroallergens. The main allergens in this category include dust mites, animal dander, and cockroaches. While outdoor plant products are dependent on climate factors for their release, the allergens that follow are often indoors and therefore nearly independent of geographical location and outdoor climate.

8.2.2 Information About Dust Mites… Lay It On Me!

Dust mites are small (0.2–0.3 mm long) arachnids (eight-legged) (▶ Fig. 8.1). Their diet includes shed human skin and fungi. Mite growth is augmented by elevated humidity. While multiple species of dust mite exist, the two most important specimens are *D. farinae* (predominates in North America) and *D. pteronyssinus* (predominates in Europe). The allergens created by dust mites are expressed in their feces, as well as their bodies. Environmental control measures aim to reduce favorable mite living conditions (humidity control) and barriers to prevent shed-skin (their food) transmission. However, it should be noted that while environmental control measures are routinely advocated

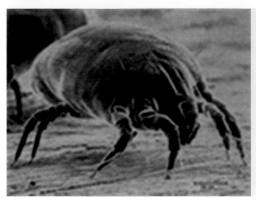

Fig. 8.1 Scanning electron microscope view of a dust mite.

in the allergy practice, the evidence of benefit is not as strong as for pharmacologic intervention or allergen immunotherapy. It often takes several different environmental control measures performed together to have an effect on allergic symptomatology related to house dust mites. As a single measure, acaricides tend to be the most beneficial.

8.2.3 What About Pet Dander?

While animal hair itself is not terribly allergenic (not buoyant nor soluble), it does carry water-soluble proteins from the epidermis or saliva, which are important. Desquamated skin (dander) can contain major allergens such as Fel d 1 from cats or Can f 1 from dogs. The dander will contain many proteins, hence these products will have major and minor allergens as well. Even pet urine and feces possess allergens. The amounts in which dogs and cats produce allergens vary; hypoallergenic pets may excrete fewer antigens, but it is not nil. Pets also vary in their production of minor antigens, which may be selectively important in patients. Cat antigens appear to be somewhat "sticky" because they persist in a home for months even after removal of a cat. Horse antigen can be potent as well, though exposure is less prevalent. Laboratory workers and animal handlers are at risk for sensitivity to rodents such as mice and rats.

8.2.4 Which Epidermals and Danders Have Major Allergens That Are Known?

The following epidermals and danders have had major allergens identified:
- Cat: Fel d 1.
- Rat: Rat n 1.
- Mouse: Mus m 1.

- Dog: Can f 1.
- Dust mites (Dp, Df): Der p 1, 2; Der f 1, 2

8.2.5 Which Epidermals and Danders Have Standard Allergen Extracts Available?

Standardized allergen extracts are available in the United States for the following epidermals and danders:

- Cat hair.
- Cat pelt.
- *Dermatophagoides farinae.*
- *Dermatophagoides pteronyssinus.*

Clinical Pearls	M!

- Perennial allergens are an important source of year-round allergy symptoms. Some of the most common perennial allergens come from dust mites, cat, and dog.
- Patients with occupational or hobby-related contact to mice and horses may also experience allergy symptoms.

Bibliography

[1] Patterson R, Grammer LC, Greenberger PA, eds. Allergic Diseases: Diagnosis and Management. New York, NY: Lippincott Williams & Wilkins; 1997
[2] Wise SK, Lin SY, Toskala E, et al. International consensus statement on allergy and rhinology: allergic rhinitis. Int Forum Allergy Rhinol. 2018; 8(2):108–352

9 Inhalant Allergens: Weeds

Steven M. Houser, Sarah K. Wise

9.1 When Weeds Are the Worst

Patients with late summer or fall allergy symptoms may be reacting to weed pollen. The primary weeds of allergenic importance in North America include the composites and chenopod-amaranths. Ragweed has several types but remains the main allergenic weed in North America.

Please see Chapter 5 for a review of the following topics:

- Definition of antigen, allergen, and epitope.
- Major versus minor allergens.
- Allergen extract units, standardized versus nonstandardized allergen extracts.
- Cross-reactivity.
- Thommen's postulates.
- Description of pollen particles and the plants that produce pollen.

9.2 Serious Stuff

9.2.1 What Are the Common Types of Allergenic Weeds in North America?

North American weeds of allergenic importance can be divided into two groups: composites and chenopod-amaranths. Other weeds may be of local importance as well.

The composite weeds (Asteraceae family) include three large tribes of common, highly allergenic weeds: Heliantheae, Anthemideae, and Astereae tribes. The Heliantheae tribe includes cocklebur, marsh elder, and ragweed. Ragweed remains the primary allergenic weed in most of North America (▶ Fig. 9.1). Multiple species of ragweed exist including false, giant, short, and western; these have been shown to strongly cross-react with one another. Short ragweed is often used as the representative for this family for testing and treatment unless the specific climate generates a different locally abundant weed.

The Anthemideae (sage) tribe contains mugwort, sagebrush, wormwood, sage, and chrysanthemum; the latter two are edible members. Mugwort is the most important weed along the Pacific coast of North America as well as in Europe. Mugwort cross-reacts approximately 80% with ragweed.

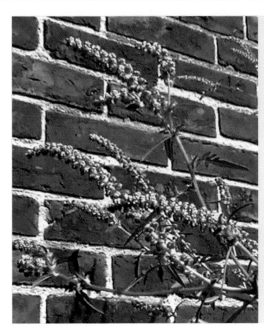

Fig. 9.1 Ragweed.

Baccharis species, aster (daisy), and goldenrod are members of the Astereae (daisy) tribe. Goldenrod is predominantly entomophilous for pollination, but sensitivities to the airborne pollen might still exist. This tribe is most important along the coastal and western United States.

Additional composite weeds may not be major sources of pollen, but rather are potent contact sensitizers. Some examples include the Cynareae tribe (e.g., thistles, artichoke) and the Cichorieae tribe (e.g., dandelion, chicory). Lettuce and stevia are additional edible members of the Asteraceae family.

The Amaranthaceae family is closely related to the Chenopodiaceae family, hence often termed the *Amaranth-Chenopods*. These weeds are very common and are major pollinators. Amaranth examples include cockscomb, careless weed, cottonweed, pigweed, water hemp, and the edible quinoa. The Chenopod family is represented by Kochia (e.g., burning bush), goosefoot, lamb's quarters, Mexican tea, and the edibles: beet, spinach, and sugar beet. The Amaranths strongly cross-react, while the Chenopods cross-react only mildly; a single Amaranth can be used for allergy testing and treatment within the family, while Chenopods usually need to be treated individually.

9.2.2 What About Minor Weed Families, or Locally Important Weeds?

Multiple minor weed families exist and they tend to be of more importance in individual locations. English plantain (Plantaginaceae family) is perhaps the most important minor weed, affecting the middle portion of North America. Sheep and dock sorrel (Polygonaceae family) are fairly common as well. The Cannabaceae family includes hemp, marijuana, hops, and hackberry that may be locally important. Lesser minor weeds include the nettles (Urticaceae family) and mustard and rape plants (Brassicaceae family).

9.2.3 What Else Should I Know About Weeds... or Weed "Imposters?"

Weed-like sporulating Pteridophytes are not weeds, but might be mistaken as such. Pteridophytes produce spores rather than flowers and seeds. These plants may be of local importance in allergic sensitization, especially in the tropics (e.g., Southeast Asia). Some examples of their unique group include ferns, horsetails, and club mosses (e.g., *Lycopodium*).

9.2.4 When Do Weeds Pollinate?

Late summer and fall is the typical season for weed pollination in North America. Allergy patients with symptoms during this time may be reacting to weed pollen aeroallergens.

9.2.5 What Are Some Common Allergenic Weeds?

The box below (Box 9.1) lists some common allergenic weeds.

Weeds (angiosperm)
  Asteraceae (Compositae) family
    Heliantheae tribe
      Ragweed, cocklebur, marshelder
    Astereae tribe
      Goldenrod, daisy, Baccharis species
    Anthemideae tribe
      Mugwort, chamomile, sagebrush, wormwood
      Sage, chrysanthemum
  Amaranthaceae family
    Amaranths, pigweed, cockscomb
    Quinoa
  Chenopodiaceae family
    Lamb's quarters, burning bush, Russian thistle
    Goosefoot, Mexican tea
    Beet, spinach, sugar beet
  Brassicaceae
    Mustard, rape
  Cannabaceae
    Hemp, marijuana, hops, hackberry
  Plantaginaceae
    English plantain
  Polygonaceae
    Dock, sorrel
  Urticeaea
    Nettles

9.2.6 Which Weeds Have Major Allergens That Are Known?

The following weeds have had major allergens identified:
- Short Ragweed: Amb a 1, 2, 3, 5, 6.
- Giant ragweed: Amb t 5.
- Mugwort: Art v 1.

9.2.7 Which Weeds Have Standard Allergen Extracts Available?

Short ragweed has standardized allergen extracts available in the United States.

Clinical Pearls **M!**

- Allergenic weeds of North America typically consist of composites and chenopod-amaranths.
- The Heliantheae tribe of composite weeds includes cocklebur, marsh elder, and ragweed. Ragweed is the primary allergenic weed in most of North America.
- Amaranths include cockscomb, careless weed, cottonweed, pigweed, and quinoa.
- The Chenopod family includes Kochia (e.g., burning bush), lamb's quarters, beet, spinach, and a few others.
- Weeds typically pollinate in the late summer and fall months.

Bibliography

[1] Hirschwehr R, Heppner C, Spitzauer S, et al. Identification of common allergenic structures in mugwort and ragweed pollen. J Allergy Clin Immunol. 1998; 101(2 Pt 1):196–206

[2] Kaplan AP, ed. Allergy. Philadelphia, PA: W.B. Saunders Company; 1997

[3] Leiferman KM, Gleich GJ, Jones RT. The cross-reactivity of IgE antibodies with pollen allergens. II. Analyses of various species of ragweed and other fall weed pollens. J Allergy Clin Immunol. 1976; 58(1 PT. 2):140–148

[4] Rodríguez A, De Barrio M, De Frutos C, de Benito V, Baeza ML. Occupational allergy to fern. Allergy. 2001; 56(1):89

Part 2

Diagnosis of Allergy

10 History

Christine B. Franzese

It's normal not to breathe through your nose.

A patient said this to me recently, and I've heard variations of this from a few other patients. Actually, it's quite normal to breathe through your nose, but I use this example to highlight the necessary peril you face when taking a patient's history to make the clinical diagnosis of allergy or allergic rhinitis. The clinical history is vital to making the diagnosis, but it's not uncommon for patients who have lived with certain symptoms for longer duration that those symptoms (such as nasal congestion or nasal obstruction) become their new "normal."

Hence many patients consider seasonal allergy symptoms or "hay fever" to be normal, that everyone has them, and may not give you those symptoms without some prompting. They may complain that they have "symptoms" (or "the sinus" or "the crud"). Needless to say, it is necessary to dig further and record what exactly these symptoms are (not just to document for billing purposes) but to help in determining the most likely diagnosis and treatment for the patient.

10.1 History of Present Illness

What are the necessary parts of the history of present illness (HPI)? Type of symptoms, timing and duration, frequency, inciting exposures, current/past medications used to treat, comorbid conditions (asthma, eczema, etc.), family history of atopy (asthma, eczema, etc.), response to any medications used consist this information.

What kind of symptoms do I look for? ▸ Table 10.1 lists general symptoms that are suggestive of allergic disease and other diseases. It is not exhaustive, encompassing, or absolute.

Table 10.1 List of symptoms

Symptoms suggestive of allergy	Symptoms suggestive of other disorders
Clear nasal drainage[a]	Discolored nasal drainage
Nasal congestion/obstruction[a]	Decreased sense of smell/taste
Sneezing/sniffing[a]	Headache/facial or sinus pain
Eye, nasal, oral, throat itching[a]	Oral or nasal masses/ulcers
Red and/or water eyes	Discolored sputum
Wheezing/coughing (dry)	

[a]These symptoms rank highest in diagnostic utility for allergic rhinitis.

Other symptoms that might suggest allergy include hyposmia/anosmia, snoring, decreased hearing/"clogged ears" due to middle ear fluid, snoring, sore throat, postnasal drip, hoarseness/throat clearing.

What about timing and symptoms? Are the symptoms year-round (perennial), seasonal, or intermittent (with exposure to an allergic trigger)?

> Patients with year-round allergies tend to report congestive symptoms (sinus pressure, nasal blockage/congestion, and snoring). Patients with season allergies are more likely to complain of sore throat, cough, sneezing, rhinorrhea, and postnasal drip.

10.2 Past Medical History

What are some allergy associated comorbid conditions? Past medical history (PMH) such as asthma, eczema, food allergy, sleep-disordered breathing or obstructive sleep apnea, otitis media (in older children) may be seen in patients with allergic disorder.

> ⚠
> It's very important to ask about other medical conditions. While not directly related to allergy, other medical conditions, such as heart disease or stroke, effect a patient's ability to survive a serious allergic reaction and must be taken into account during any discussion of treatment.

10.3 Past Surgical History

Why are surgeries relevant here? Certain surgical procedures may indicate associated allergic comorbid conditions. Myringotomy tubes, adenotonsillectomy, and inferior turbinate reduction are important procedures to anticipate while treating allergy patient.

10.4 Medications

Why is this necessary? A list of current medications, including over-the-counter medications, vitamins, and herbal remedies, is necessary as certain medications (including herbal remedies) can impact allergy testing. See Chapter 14 for further details.

> It's not uncommon for patients to leave off medication(s) they use to control allergy symptoms, even if taken daily. Be sure to ask about them.

10.5 Family/Social History

Does family history matter? Yes. Certain allergic disorders have a hereditary component(s). Be sure to ask about any family members with allergies, asthma, etc.

What's important about social history? Be sure to ask about environmental and occupational exposures. Ask about any pets, farm animals, and exposure to tobacco smoke.

10.6 Review of Systems

Why is this important? Frequently, patients will have undiagnosed comorbid conditions. It's not uncommon for patients to have frequent cough/wheezing, have an albuterol inhaler, but not have a diagnosis of reactive airway disease or asthma in their medical history. This area is helpful to catch any potential undiagnosed medical conditions that may affect diagnostic workup or treatment plan.

Clinical Pearls   M!

- The diagnosis of allergy is frequently made on the basis of history alone.
- Types of symptoms, timing, exposures, and other parts of the history can give information that is suggestive of allergy or alert the immunologist to check for other potential nonallergic diagnoses.

Bibliography

[1] Schatz M. A survey of the burden of allergic rhinitis in the USA. Allergy. 2007; 62 Suppl 85:9–16
[2] Ng ML, Warlow RS, Chrishanthan N, Ellis C, Walls R. Preliminary criteria for the definition of allergic rhinitis: a systematic evaluation of clinical parameters in a disease cohort (I). Clin Exp Allergy. 2000; 30(9):1314–1331
[3] Costa DJ, Amouyal M, Lambert P, et al. Languedoc-Roussillon Teaching General Practitioners Group. How representative are clinical study patients with allergic rhinitis in primary care? J Allergy Clin Immunol. 2011; 127(4):920–6.e1

11 Patient Surveys and Questionnaires

Christine B. Franzese

11.1 To Use or Not to Use

Yes, that's a question. As in, what use do patient surveys and questionnaires have in actual clinical practice? Sure, their use in research makes sense, and maybe even in academic practice, but if you're in a busy private practice, you may dismiss these out of hand has having little to no utility and skip this chapter. This chapter explains how these instruments can be used effectively. Does author use these instruments while treating patients? Yes. Does the author get useful information from them? Most of the time. Do they cause problems? Yes, because patients complain about having to fill them out.

While discussing these types of surveys and questionnaires, only those instruments validated by the literature have been mentioned in this chapter. The author is not referring to a patient questionnaire that is available in every practice asking for various bits of information that help the practitioner with history taking. These validated instruments do have their place in actual clinical practice and can be useful in measuring and documenting patient outcomes.

11.2 The Basics

What is a patient-reported outcome measures (PROMs)? A patient-reported outcome is a health outcome that a patient directly reports, and the measure is the method that is used to capture that information. These measures include questionnaires, such as quality-of-life (QoL) questionnaires and surveys.

What is a QoL questionnaire? This is a clinically validated questionnaire that measures the relationship between the patient's QoL (or certain aspects of QoL) and other behaviors, symptoms, or disease processes.

What's a survey? And what's the difference between a survey and a questionnaire? The technical definition of a survey is a process for gathering data that may involve different types of data collection methods, including a questionnaire. It's a much broader term than questionnaire. A questionnaire is an instrument asking a given a set of oral or written questions. With the instruments given in ▶ Table 11.1, in the author's opinion, there is not much difference between a "survey" and a "questionnaire." These two terms are used interchangeably in this chapter.

Which one should the practitioner use? Each instrument measures different things and has its own strengths and weaknesses. Some popular instruments are listed in ▶ Table 11.1 to help the practitioner decide what to use. Some ideas are also given on how to effectively use them and avoid patient complaints.

Table 11.1 The instruments

Name of instrument	No. of questions	What it measures (Pro[s])	Con(s)
Global Assessment of Severity of Allergy	1	Severity of rhinitis (easy and quick)	Not much other information
Total Nasal Symptom Score	4	Symptoms score at that moment in time (easy and quick)	No medication usage information, only one point in time
Allergic Rhinitis Control Test	5	Symptoms and medication usage (quick)	Limited information, only covers allergic rhinitis
Rhinitis Control Assessment Test	6	Symptoms of rhinitis (quick)	No medication usage, only analyze rhinitis control
Rhinoconjunctivitis Allergy Control Score	7 + meds	Symptoms plus medications	No questions on asthma, not as quick
Symptom Score For Allergic Rhinitis	8	More information on symptoms	No medication usage, not as quick
Allergy Control Score	10 + meds	Medication usage and symptoms	Not as quick, includes asthma
Mini-Rhinoconjunctivitis QoL Questionnaire	14	More information on symptoms (over a week)	No medication usage information, not as fast
Rhinoconjunctivitis QoL Questionnaire	28	Details information on symptoms over a week	No medication usage, recall bias, longer time

Abbreviation: QoL, Quality of Life.

11.3 My Humble Suggestions

Where to get these? Some are available on the Internet at various Web sites. Some of them require permission to use, some don't. Some are posted that are adapted for use in other practices. The most important thing is to decide what to measure and why. This will help in determining which tool to use. From there, quick search on the Internet will get you want what. Be sure to get permission where it is needed.

Where these can be useful? They can help to objectively assess severity of symptoms and amount of medication used. They can be used to show patients (or demonstrate outcomes) improvement of symptoms/medication usage. There are times when patients may have been on therapy for a while and become forgetful of exactly how bad their condition was before starting immunotherapy. These can show patients the difference between where they were and where they are now.

Where these can cause problems? When too many surveys are used. When different surveys that measure the same things are used together. When they are used too frequently. When they are longer. When they are not available in languages other than English. When they contain complex terminology rather than simple language or pictures.

Pick one (maybe two) and stick with that. Administer the instrument(s) at the initial visit, then on a yearly basis. If the form can be entered directly into note or the electronic medical record (EMR), even better. If not, then in addition to scanning the form in, have your nurse enter the score within your note. That way you can look back in your notes to find previous scores, without having to resort to pulling up scanned documents.

Clinical Pearls M!

- Questionnaires and patient surveys are an easy way to demonstrate patient-outcome improvement.
- Too many questionnaires and/or too frequent administration causes problems.
- Pick one. Use it on the initial visit, then yearly thereafter.

Bibliography

[1] Calderon MA, Bernstein DI, Blaiss M, Andersen JS, Nolte H. A comparative analysis of symptom and medication scoring methods used in clinical trials of sublingual immunotherapy for seasonal allergic rhinitis. Clin Exp Allergy. 2014; 44(10):1228–1239

[2] Devillier P, Bousquet PJ, Grassin-Delyle S, et al. Comparison of outcome measures in allergic rhinitis in children, adolescents and adults. Pediatr Allergy Immunol. 2016; 27(4):375–381

12 Physical Examination

Christine B. Franzese

12.1 Not All That Sniffles Is Allergic

A physician may be tempted to overlook the physical examination of an allergic patient, but it's an important part of your workup. Yes, it is true that frequently the physical examination can be completely normal. However, that's no reason to skip this part or do a cursory examination. While it is helpful to discover findings suggestive of allergy, one of the main reasons to do a thorough physical examination is to discover those findings that suggest it's *not* allergy (or at least, *not only* allergy). It's disheartening to both patient and provider when the patient, who has undergone immunotherapy for an extended period of time, perceives little to no benefit, because he/she is suffering from another medical condition (chronic sinusitis, nasal polyposis, etc.). The physical examination isn't necessarily important because it helps you diagnose allergic disease, but because it helps you diagnose or eliminate other disorders.

12.2 The Physical

What are you looking for? ▶ Table 12.1 provides a general guide and includes physical examination findings that are suggestive if the patient is suffering from allergic disease or not. It is not exhaustive, encompassing, or absolute (▶ Fig. 12.1, ▶ Fig. 12.2, ▶ Fig. 12.3, ▶ Fig. 12.4).

Table 12.1 Physical examination findings

Physical examination area	Suggestive of allergy	Suggestive of other disorders
Eye (▶ Fig. 12.1)	Conjunctival erythema/edema Watery discharge Periorbital edema "Allergic shiners": Dark discoloration of lower lids/periorbital area	Discolored discharge Change in vision Light sensitivity Absence of pupillary reflex
Ear	Retracted tympanic membrane Clear middle ear effusion	Bulging tympanic membrane Purulent/opaque middle ear effusion Perforation

Table 12.1 (*continued*)

Physical examination area	Suggestive of allergy	Suggestive of other disorders
Nose (anterior rhinoscopy/nasal endoscopy) (▶ Fig. 12.2, ▶ Fig. 12.3, ▶ Fig. 12.4)	Supratip nasal crease Clear nasal drainage Bluish/purplish nasal mucosa Inferior turbinate hypertrophy	Discolored/purulent nasal drainage Erythematous nasal mucosa Middle turbinate enlargement Nasal polyps/mass Enlarged adenoids
Oral cavity/pharynx	Cobblestoning of pharyngeal mucosa Lateral pharyngeal bands Mouth breathing (adult)	Enlarged tonsils Oral/pharyngeal mass Mouth breathing (child)
Larynx (indirect mirror/direct flexible)	Stringy bridging mucus Mild edema of true vocal cords	Erythema/white plaques on true vocal cords Lesion/mass Inspiratory stridor
Lungs	Expiratory wheezing (sibilant wheeze) Nonproductive coughing	Rhonci (sonorous wheeze) Rales/crackles

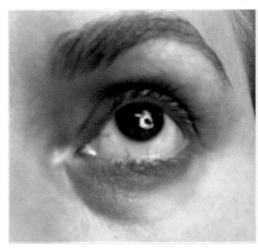

Fig. 12.1 Left eye with "allergic shiner" underneath lower eyelid.

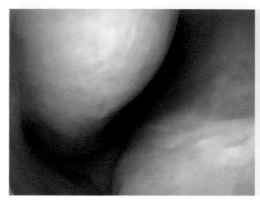

Fig. 12.2 Right enlarged inferior turbinate. Bluish discoloration of mucosa is typical of that seen with allergic rhinitis.

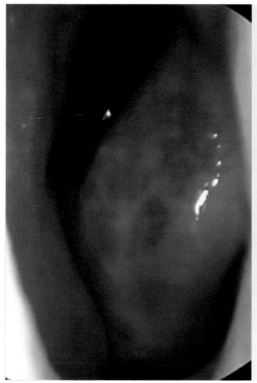

Fig. 12.3 Left enlarged inferior turbinate. Note the mixed erythematous and bluish mucosa. The erythema shown here is more typical of non-allergic rhinitis and a mixed rhinitis is pictured here.

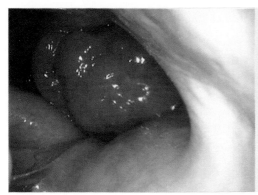

Fig. 12.4 Endoscopic view of right posterior nasopharynx. Note the enlarged adenoids and clear nasal drainage flowing over the right eustachian tube. This is typical of allergic rhinitis.

Clinical Pearls	M!

- The physical examination is important.
- Pay close attention to findings that indicate associated comorbid diseases other than allergy.

Bibliography

[1] Seidman MD, Gurgel RK, Lin SY, et al. Clinical practice guideline: allergic rhinitis executive summary. Otolaryngol Head Neck Surg. 2015; 152(2):197–206

[2] Wallace DV, Dykewicz MS, Bernstein DI, et al. Joint Task Force on Practice, American Academy of Allergy, Asthma & Immunology, American College of Allergy, Asthma and Immunology, Joint Council of Allergy, Asthma and Immunology. The diagnosis and management of rhinitis: an updated practice parameter. J Allergy Clin Immunol. 2008; 122(2) Suppl:S1–S84

13 Differential Diagnosis

Christine B. Franzese

"Doc, I got the sinus"

Allergic rhinitis is a very common disorder and frequently patients will have their own euphemisms to describe the symptoms of allergies. While practicing in Mississippi, it was not unusual for a patient to tell the author that he/she had "the sinus," not meaning a sinus infection, but actually referring to the sensation of sinus pressure, nasal congestion, and sneezing associated with an allergic flare-up. Allergies aren't always to blame, though, and there are some equally common, nonallergic causes for nasal symptoms similar to those associated with allergic rhinitis.

13.1 The Mimics and Imposters

Here are some of the most common mimics of allergic rhinitis:

Viral rhinitis: Frequently confused with allergic rhinitis, viral rhinitis tends to last 4 to 6 days and is associated with the sneezing, clear nasal drainage, and nasal congestion that is typical of allergies. Fever can be helpful to distinguish this from allergies, but often may not occur, particularly in adults. Sore throat doesn't help distinguish a viral infection from allergies.

Age-related (senile) rhinitis: The process of aging with its decline in autonomic function can lead to vasodilation and increased mucus consistency and quantity, resulting in nasal congestion and clear drainage that can appear similar to allergy. Complaints of clear nasal drainage actually increase with age, but true allergic rhinitis decreases as a person ages, due to changes in immune functions.

Nonallergic/vasomotor rhinitis: Inflammation is not a part of this type of rhinitis, which is the most common cause of nonallergic causes of rhinitis. This is a diagnosis of exclusion, tends to be more common in females than males, and the nasal mucosa look erythematous on physical examination.

> Beware of the migraine patient. Patients with a history of migraines will frequently neglect to tell you about their migraines (or haven't been properly diagnosed yet). Migraine sufferers can frequently develop a sinus pressure "headache" that may be accompanied by nasal congestion and runny nose, but it won't respond very well to allergy medications. It generally will respond to migraine medications.

Drug-induced rhinitis: Certain systemic medications can cause local inflammatory and neurogenic effects to the nasal mucosa that induce rhinitis. Some common medications associated with rhinitis are:

- Nonsteroidal anti-inflammatory drugs (NSAIDS), antihypertensives such as beta blockers, vasodilators, immunosuppressants, psychotropics, alpha blockers, presynaptic alpha agonists, phosphodiesterase (PDE)-5 specific inhibitors, PDE-3 and nonselective PDE inhibitors, and angiotensin converting enzyme (ACE) inhibitors. Illicit use of both illegal and legal prescription drugs taken via a nasal route can also induce chronic rhinitis.

Rhinitis medicamentosa: A drug-induced rhinitis that deserves special mention. Caused by prolonged use of intranasal decongestants and associated with rebound congestion and rhinitis, the patient may not always disclose using these medications or may think that "this is the only medication that makes me better."

Chemical/irritant rhinitis: This may occur with or without occupational exposures and includes both high- and low-molecular-weight agents.

- Some examples of occupations with associated chemical or irritant exposures include bakers/food preparation workers (flour), health care workers (latex, pharmaceutical agents), hair dressers (persulphates), pharmaceutical/detergent industrial workers (biologic agents/enzymes), carpenters/craftsmen (wood dust), and cleaners/chemical industrial workers (chemical irritants).
- Some examples of nonoccupational activities associated with chemical or irritant exposures include swimming (chlorine), cleaning (ammonia, chemicals), and wearing new clothes (formaldehyde).

Rhinitis of pregnancy/hormonal rhinitis: This tends to start after 8 to 10 weeks of pregnancy, get worse in the second trimester, and spontaneously resolves within 2 weeks of delivery. It is difficult to treat, generally not responsive to allergy medications including intranasal steroids, and may improve with hypertonic nasal saline rinses.

Clinical Pearls M!

- Look for specific triggers to help determine if symptoms are due to allergies or another cause.
- None of these mimics demonstrate type 1 immunoglobulin (IgE)-mediated hypersensitivity.
- Allergies tend to decrease with age, be sure to evaluate for senile rhinitis.
- Some mimics will respond to certain types of allergy medications, but others won't.

Bibliography

[1] Dykewicz MS, Fineman S, Skoner DP, et al. Diagnosis and management of rhinitis: complete guidelines of the Joint Task Force on Practice Parameters in Allergy, Asthma and Immunology. American Academy of Allergy, Asthma, and Immunology. Ann Allergy Asthma Immunol. 1998; 81 (5 Pt 2):478–518

[2] Quillen DM, Feller DB. Diagnosing rhinitis: allergic vs. nonallergic. Am Fam Physician. 2006; 73 (9):1583–1590

[3] Siracusa A, Folletti I, Moscato G. Non-IgE-mediated and irritant-induced work-related rhinitis. Curr Opin Allergy Clin Immunol. 2013; 13(2):159–166

Part 3

Testing Methods

14 Conditions That Can Impact Skin Testing

Christine B. Franzese

14.1 Setting the Stage for Success

Once the decision has been made to proceed with diagnostic testing, the next decision point is *what type* of allergy testing should be performed. While this book covers both skin testing and serum-specific immunoglobulin (IgE) testing ("blood" testing), only skin testing requires some candidate selection and preparation. Certain medical conditions or medications (with the exception of omalizumab) do not influence serum-specific IgE testing. In this chapter common conditions and medications that impact skin testing are discussed.

14.2 Medical Conditions

Dermatographism: The most common type of physical urticaria, resulting when a wheal and flare response appears when the skin is scratched or scraped. Due to the fact that this disorder makes skin reactivity unpredictable, patients with dermatographism should undergo serum-specific IgE testing.

Dermatitis (contact, eczema, etc.): Active skin inflammation of any kind is a contraindication to skin testing if it is occurring at the site(s) where testing will be performed. In addition, frequent use of topical steroid negatively affects the accuracy of skin testing, so testing should not be performed at sites where the patient uses topical steroids.

Asthma (poorly controlled, uncontrolled): While asthma itself is not a contraindication to skin testing, poorly controlled or uncontrolled asthma increases the risk of a serious adverse reaction during the procedure. Thus, before performing any skin testing, asthma patients should be assessed for level of control both subjectively, by history, and more objectively, by spirometry, peak flow meter, or fractional exhaled nitric oxide (FeNO) testing. If the patient is poorly controlled or uncontrolled, the decision should be made to either call the patient back once the asthma is controlled or to send he/she for another type of testing.

Pregnancy: With certain, select exceptions, skin testing should not be performed in a pregnant patient.

Other serious comorbid medical conditions: While these conditions may not directly impact the wheal and flare reaction, serious medical conditions such as a history of heart attack, stroke, peripheral vascular disease, etc., may impact the patient's chance of surviving a serious adverse reaction. Any patient who has one or more serious medical condition(s) that would potentially reduce the chance of surviving a serious adverse reaction should be sent for specific IgE or other type of testing.

14.3 Medications

Certain medications affect skin testing: These consist H1-antihistamines, H2-antihistamines, certain tricyclic antidepressants, topical corticosteroids (chronic usage), and omalizumab.

Certain medications might affect skin testing: These consist benzodiazepines, topical calcineurin inhibitors, herbal remedies, and vitamin supplements.

Certain medications do not affect skin testing: These consist systemic oral corticosteroids, inhaled or intranasal steroids, leukotriene receptor antagonists, and selective serotonin reuptake inhibitors.

Other medications may affect skin testing, but haven't been adequately studied.

This disclaimer can be included on the list of medications to stop and NOT to stop. A list should be given to the patient that shows not only what medications to stop and when to stop prior to testing, but what medications they should NOT stop.

▶ Table 14.1 shows medications that can affect skin testing and when a patient should stop them. If the patient is discontinuing a medication, he/she should be advised verbally and in writing to seek the advice of the prescribing physician before discontinuing *any* medication.

Table 14.1 Medications that affect skin testing and when to discontinue them

Medication type	Days to stop prior to test
H1-antihistamines (oral): Loratadine, desloratadine, cetirizine, levocetirizine, fexofenadine	5–7 days
H1-antihistamines (oral and topical): Meclizine, diphenhydramine, azelastine, olopatadine, hydroxyzine, cyproheptadine, brompheniramine, chlorpheniramine, phenyltoloxamine, promethazine, pyrilamine	2–3 days
H2-antihistamines: Ranitidine, famotidine, cimetidine	3–4 days
Antidepressants: Doxepin	5–7 days
Antidepressants: Amitriptyline, mirtazapine, nortriptyline, desipramine, imipramine, Trazodone	3–4 days
Anti-IgE: Omalizumab	8 weeks
Benzodiazepines: Clonazepam, diazepam, lorazepam, midazolam	5–7 days
Topical corticosteroids: Hydrocortisone, triamcinolone, betamethasone, clobetasol, fluocinonide, others	2–3 weeks
Consider stopping: Vitamins and herbal remedies such as butterbur, stinging nettle, citrus unshiu powder, lycopus lucidus, spirulina, cellulose powder, traditional Chinese medicine, Indian ayurvedic medicine	5–7 days

It can be helpful to include brand names on your medication handout so that patients don't mistakenly take something they shouldn't. For example, pyrilamine is in Pamprin Multisystem Menstrual Pain relief and could be accidently missed by female patients.

14.4 Author's Experience

The author has noted that sometimes certain medications prove to be trouble makers while skin testing. These medications haven't been studied enough to make evidence-based recommendations about avoiding them, but having a discussion with patients about stopping them prior to skin testing is advisable. The two main medications are the generic formulation of topiramate and gabapentin. While the brand names of these two drugs have never appeared to affect skin tests, the generic forms periodically have.

14.5 A Special Word About Beta-Blockers

Beta-blockers are considered a relative contraindication to skin testing, mainly because they are a risk factor for more serious adverse reactions and treatment-resistant anaphylaxis. However, there are some studies that have evaluated skin testing in patients on beta-blockers and found no increase in severity or incidence of adverse reactions. This relative contraindication does not apply to testing for hypersensitivity of venomous stinging insect. The risks and benefits of skin testing should be weighed and discussed with a patient on beta-blockers, if a decision is made to proceed.

Clinical Pearls   **M!**

- Be sure to review patient's medical conditions before selecting candidates for skin testing.
- Review patient medication lists before scheduling skin testing and discuss which one(s), if any, to stop.
- Giving a list of medications (brand name, generic name, and over-the-counter) to stop before testing and the timing of when to stop proves to be helpful to patients.

Bibliography

[1] AAOA Clinical Care Statement: Medications to avoid before allergy skin testing. Available at http://www.aaoallergy.org/wp-content/uploads/2017/05/2015-Clinical-Care-Statements-Medicines-to-Avoid-Before-Allergy-Skin-Testing.pdf. Accessed December 1, 2017

[2] Bernstein IL, Li JT, Bernstein DI, et al. American Academy of Allergy, Asthma and Immunology, American College of Allergy, Asthma and Immunology. Allergy diagnostic testing: an updated practice parameter. Ann Allergy Asthma Immunol. 2008; 100(3) Suppl 3:S1–S148

15 Skin Testing: Prick

Christine B. Franzese

15.1 Most Interesting Information

Prick testing is the workhorse of allergy testing. It is commonly done without needles and (relatively) pain-free. It's also technique-dependent and does require some practice to do correctly. It requires enough pressure to indent the skin and cause micro-tears in the epidermis to allow some penetration of the allergen. However, the pressure shouldn't be enough to cause any bleeding or any significant pain. Regardless of which type of prick-test device is being used, no red blood cells should be released and no patient should be loudly vocalizing expressions of pain. This is definitely one area where less is more.

15.2 Serious Stuff

15.2.1 Who's a Good Candidate for Skin Testing?

Anyone with symptoms suggestive of immunoglobulin E (IgE)-mediated allergic disease, who doesn't have any medical contraindications listed in Chapter 14, and who is not taking any interfering medications.

15.2.2 What Does This Test Tell Me?

This test tells whether or not IgE is present to (an) antigen(s). These tests are not perfect and are technique-dependent. It does not tell you if a patient has allergy (see Chapter 3).

15.2.3 How Long Does This Test Take? When Can I Read This Test?

After applying the test to the patient's skin, a practitioner should wait for 20 minutes, although there may be some variation in that timing among practitioners. Some might wait for only 15 minutes. The author waits for 20 minutes. Then the test results can be read as either positive or negative.

15.2.4 What Is a Positive Test? What Does It Tell Me?

A positive test is growth of a wheal of 3 mm or greater than the negative control. Generally, a positive-test result confirms the presence of IgE to (an) antigen(s). A positive test by itself only indicates allergen sensitization, NOT allergy.

15.2.5 What Is a Negative Test? What Does It Tell Me?

A negative test shows no growth or growth of a wheal less than 3 mm greater than the negative control. Generally, a negative-test result indicates the absence of IgE to (an) antigen(s).

15.2.6 What's This Negative Control and What's a Wheal?

One thing at a time! The negative control is whatever liquid the antigen concentrate is suspended in. For some company's antigens, that's 50% glycerin so you would use 50% glycerin as the negative control. For others, it may be human serum albumen (HAS) or another solution. Whatever that solution is will be what your negative control is. In the US, most commonly antigen companies use 50% glycerin in their concentrate vials. In that case, the negative control would be 50% glycerin.

15.2.7 And the Wheal?

It's the palpable induration in the skin. Its size is measured and recorded. In the past, the size of the wheal was rated between 1 and 4, but that sort of grading scale is not recommended. Record the size of the wheal in millimeters.

15.2.8 Do You Need a Positive and Negative Control? Why?

Yes, because the practitioner needs to make sure the skin reacts as expected. The practitioner needs to confirm that it will react to histamine appropriately and won't react to other things. See Chapter 14.

15.2.9 What's the Positive Control?

The positive control is histamine (6 mg/mL) for percutaneous testing. There are different concentrations of histamine made for different types of testing. Make sure to use the correct concentration (▶ Fig. 15.1).

15.2.10 What Antigens Do I Test for?

See Chapters 5 to 9. A practitioner should tailor tests according to the patient and include any relevant exposures (i.e., if the patient has a guinea pig or works in a research lab with rats, etc.).

15.2.11 Where Do I Test?

Generally, this test is done in the office. But a practitioner can perform this test at other locations as long as he/she is prepared to handle possible anaphylaxis.

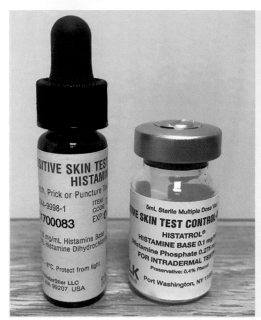

Fig. 15.1 Different types of histamines **(a)** for prick testing, **(b)** for intradermal testing.

15.2.12 No, I Mean, Where on the Patient Do I Place These Tests?

Most commonly the volar surface of the forearm, arm, and back are used.

15.2.13 Could Anaphylaxis Really Happen During Skin-Prick Testing?

Yes! It's rare and unlikely to happen, but patients may experience a variety of adverse events while testing. See Chapters 34 and 35 for allergy emergencies or urgencies, but a practitioner must be prepared to handle anaphylaxis while performing any form of skin testing.

15.2.14 Tools of the Trade (What You'll Need)

▸ Fig. 15.2 shows tools used for skin testing.
- Skin testing device (single- or multi-prick device).
- Alcohol swabs or 70% isopropyl alcohol/gloves/skin marker/record sheet or electronic medical record (EMR) entry.
- Histamine for percutaneous skin testing.

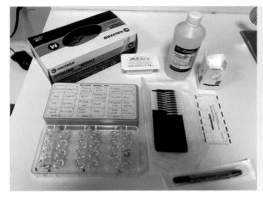

Fig. 15.2 Supplies for prick testing, both single and multi-test.

- Negative control (50% glycerin if glycerinated antigen; use whatever solution the antigen is in).
- Antigen with or without Dipwell or Tray.
- Emergency supplies (see Chapters 34 and 35).
- Wheal measuring device.

15.3 Shocking Information (How to Actually Do This!)

Verify the following points with the patient:
- Have they discontinued any interfering medications?
- Are they feeling well (not sick)?
- Have asthmatic patients suffered any recent exacerbations/rescue medication usage?
- Is the patient pregnant?

If you have a spirometer in your clinic it is helpful to perform spirometry on suspected or known asthmatic patients prior to testing.

15.4 Single Prick Device Technique

15.4.1 Step 1

Clean the area of skin being tested with an alcohol swab and allow area to dry (▶ Fig. 15.3).

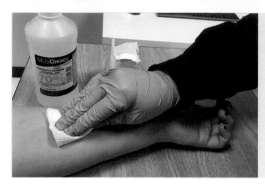

Fig. 15.3 Cleaning patient's skin with 70% isopropyl alcohol.

15.4.2 Step 2

If the Skin Prick Device (SPD) is not placed in a Dipwell or in a tray filled with antigen, then put a small droplet of antigen on skin.

If the antigen vial doesn't have a dropper, it's helpful to use an insulin or Tuberculin (TB) syringe to remove a tiny amount of antigen from the vial, then discard the needle and use the needless syringe to place a droplet or two on the patient's skin (▶ Fig. 15.4a, b).

15.4.3 Step 3

Tense the skin by using nondominant hand. Then following the manufacturer's recommended technique for the device that is being used, apply pressure to the device so that it indents the skin (▶ Fig. 15.5a, b; ▶ Fig. 15.6a, b). If the antigen drop is already on the skin, press the device through the droplet. If the device was in a Dipwell, a droplet of antigen will remain behind on the skin.

Check antigen levels in the Dipwell regularly! If the Dipwell is underfilled, not enough antigen will get on the device leading to possible inaccurate test results.

Note: NO BLEEDING! NO BRUISING! ▶ Fig. 15.7 shows examples of proper and improper technique.

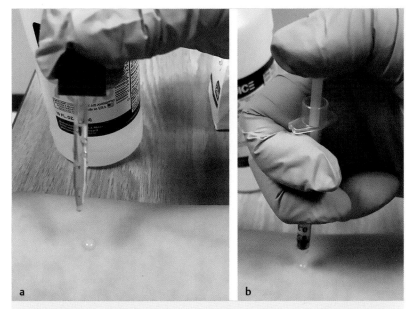

Fig. 15.4 (a) Using a dropper to place antigen on skin. **(b)** Using a needless syringe to place antigen on skin.

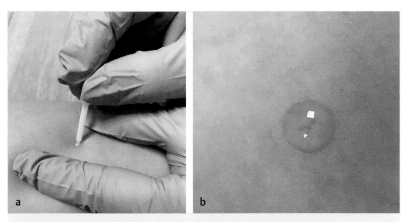

Fig. 15.5 (a) Single prick test technique. **(b)** When properly performed, the indentation left behind from the device can be seen but there is no bleeding.

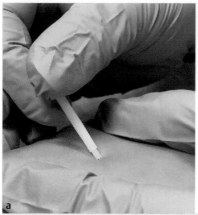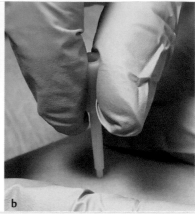

Fig. 15.6 (a) Prick testing done with the device angled at 45 degrees to the skin.
(b) Prick testing done with the device angled at 90 degrees to the skin.

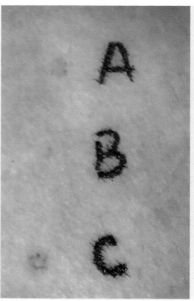

Fig. 15.7 A is correct amount of pressure on device. **B** is too little pressure—note indentation is very faint. **C** is too much pressure—note the intense outline left. This hurt a lot, bled, then bruised.

15.4.4 Step 4

Be sure to apply tests at least 2 cm apart from each other. This prevents cross-contamination and false-positives from large spreading wheals.

15.4.5 Step 5

Once all tests are applied, entertain the patient for 20 minutes. Be sure to have a television or other video entertainment device in the waiting room so that patients do not get bored before the test can be read. An allergy nurse with good people skills who might chat with the patient is a good option as well.

15.4.6 Step 6

Using a measuring device, measure each wheal and record it. The "wheal" that is being measured is the raised induration of the skin (not the redness of the skin, which is called the "flare") (▶ Fig. 15.8 and ▶ Fig. 15.9).

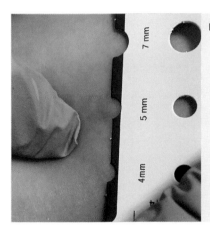

Fig. 15.8 Measuring the wheal.

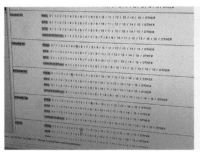

Fig. 15.9 Recording wheal sizes in millimeters in an electronic medical record (EMR).

> It is very helpful to palpate the wheal and tense the skin to make it easier to see for measurement.

15.4.7 Step 7

At this point, the patient should still have a pulse and respirations. Congratulations! The next challenge you face is to determine what you do with the test results. Good luck with that.

15.5 Multi-Prick Device Technique

15.5.1 Step 1

Clean the area of skin being tested with an alcohol swab and allow the area to dry (see ▶ Fig. 15.3).

15.5.2 Step 2

Place multi-test device(s) in a Dipwell tray. Remove device when you are ready to apply it to the patient's skin.

> Check antigen levels in the Dipwell regularly! If the Dipwell is underfilled, not enough antigen will get on the device leading to possible inaccurate test results.

15.5.3 Step 3

Tense the skin by using nondominant hand and following the manufacturer's recommended technique for the device that is being used, apply pressure to the device such that it indents the skin (▶ Fig. 15.10a, b).

> NO BLEEDING! NO BRUISING! (▶ Fig. 15.11)

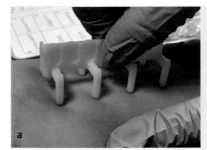

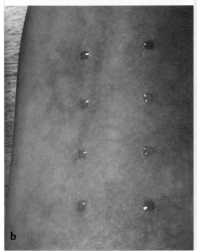

Fig. 15.10 (a) Multi-test device technique. **(b)** With proper pressure all the indentations are seen at each site, but no bleeding.

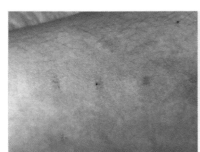

Fig. 15.11 Too much pressure—blood, pain. Ouch!

15.5.4 Step 4

When applying more than one device, be sure to separate the device applications by at least 2 cm (▶ Fig. 15.12).

15.5.5 Step 5

Once all tests are applied, entertain yourself and/or the patient for 20 minutes (▶ Fig. 15.13).

15.5.6 Step 6

Using a measuring device, measure each wheal and record it. The "wheal" that is being measured is the raised induration of the skin (not the redness of the skin, which is called the "flare").

It is helpful to palpate the wheal and tense the skin to make it easier to see for measurement (▶ Fig. 15.14).

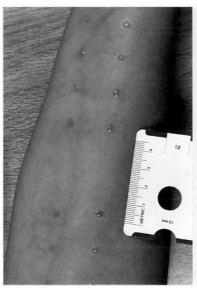

Fig. 15.12 Make sure there's enough space between different testing panels.

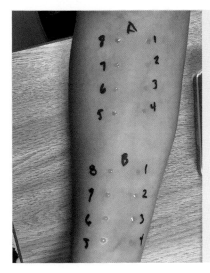

Fig. 15.13 Be sure to mark the testing panels after application.

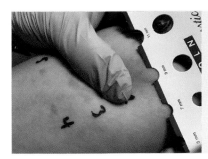

Fig. 15.14 Measuring the wheal size. Note how tensing the skin makes the wheal easier to see.

15.5.7 Step 7

At this point, the patient should still have a pulse and respirations. Congratulations! Now you have to figure out what you're going to do with the information you've gleaned from this test. Good luck with that.

Clinical Pearls

M!

- The practitioner should have the knowledge about the device that is being used, and the manufacturer's recommended technique for it.
- Use the correct positive and negative controls.
- NO BLEEDING!
- Read test at 20 minutes.
  - A positive test is wheal growth of 3 mm or greater than the negative control.
  - A negative test is no wheal growth or growth less than 3 mm or greater than the negative control.
  - Allergy = History + Positive test result. A positive test by itself only indicates sensitization.
  - Be prepared to handle anaphylaxis.

Bibliography

[1] Berstein, et al. "Allergy diagnostic testing: an updated practice parameter." Available at https://www.aaaai.org/Aaaai/media/MediaLibrary/PDF%20Documents/Practice%20and%20Parameters/allergydiagnostictesting.pdf. Accessed October 1, 2017

[2] King HC, Mabry RL, Gordon BR, et al. Allergy in ENT Practice: The Basic Guide. Thieme; 2004

[3] Nevis IF, Binkley K, Kabali C. Diagnostic accuracy of skin-prick testing for allergic rhinitis: a systematic review and meta-analysis. Allergy Asthma Clin Immunol. New York, NY: Thieme; 2016; 12:20

16 Skin Testing: Intradermal

Christine B. Franzese

16.1 Getting into (not under) Someone's Skin

Intradermal testing is another skin testing technique that can be used to diagnose allergies, either alone as a single intradermal test, together with skin prick testing (see Chapter 17 on blended techniques), or in a sequential fashion to determine a potential suggested point for immunotherapy or as done with testing for venomous stinging insect allergy. It is also used in conjunction with skin prick testing as part of the testing technique to evaluate patients with some medication allergies, such as penicillin or local anesthetic allergies. This technique involves needles, is more technique-dependent so more skill and experience are needed in placing these tests, and can cause mild discomfort. Like skin prick testing, there should be little to no bleeding and, though the risk of severe allergic reactions is slightly elevated, anaphylaxis is rare. Even if the practitioner chooses not to practice this type of skin testing, it's still helpful to be familiar with it, especially if he/she chooses to pursue adding testing for venoms or medication in the future.

16.2 Serious Stuff

Who's a good candidate for skin testing? As with skin prick testing, patients with symptoms suggestive of immunoglobulin E (IgE)-mediated allergic disease, having no medical contraindications listed in Chapter 14, and who have discontinued any interfering medications.

What does this test tell? Whether or not IgE is present to (an) antigen(s). These tests are not perfect, require more skill to perform than skin prick testing, and are technique-dependent. It does not tell if a patient has allergy (see Chapter 3). The evidence doesn't support a clear demonstration of superiority of skin prick testing over single or sequential intradermal techniques and vice versa.

How does this test differ from skin prick testing? What is the technique? Instead of an applicator device, a special short beveled needle is used to inject a tiny amount of fluid into the intradermal layer of the skin, similar to a purified protein derivative (PPD) test for tuberculosis. Roughly 0.01 to 0.03 mL of fluid is used to raise a 4-mm wheal. The testing procedure is discussed in more detail in this chapter.

What fluid is used for injection? Fluids used for injection are either the prepared positive, negative, and if indicated, glycerin controls, as well as one or more diluted preparations of antigen. What dilutions of antigen are used, as well as how to prepare them and the controls, are discussed later in the chapter.

How long does this test take? When can this test be read? After injection, wait for 10 minutes, although there may be some variation in that timing among practitioners. Then the test results can be read as either positive or negative and the wheal sizes can be recorded.

What is a negative test? What does it tell? Physical spreading of the injected fluid alone will cause enlargement of the wheal usually by 1 mm so a negative test will measure 5 mm wheal size at 10 minutes. It indicates the absence of sensitivity.

What is a positive test? What does it tell? A positive test is growth of the wheal beyond what would be expected from physical spreading alone by at least 2 mm. So a positive test would show a growth of the wheal to at least 7 mm or greater than the negative control. The exception to this is if a glycerin control is used and there is a positive result for that test. In that case, a positive test is at least 7 mm and at least 2 mm larger than the wheal produced from the glycerin control. Generally, a positive test result confirms the presence of IgE to (an) antigen(s). A positive test by itself only indicates allergen sensitization, NOT allergy.

What's the negative control? And what's a glycerin control? Why would you need that? Intradermal testing is a little bit more complicated. As mentioned before, different dilutions of antigens may be used in this testing. The negative control is whatever liquid the antigen concentrate is being diluted in, generally phenolated normal saline (PNS).

The glycerin control is basically one or more diluted preparations of 50% glycerin. Remember—each antigen concentrate contains 50% glycerin and diluting those down will create solutions with different concentrations of glycerin. In patients with glycerin sensitivity, a wheal and flare response can occur if the injected dilution contains a high amount of glycerin concentration to irritate their skin. Without a glycerin control to let you know the patient being tested has glycerin sensitivity, antigen testing reactions may be read as falsely positive.

So, can the glycerine be used or the test results can be read if the patient has a positive glycerin control? And what dilution of glycerin should be used? Yes! If the patient has a positive glycerin control, test results can be read, only the alteration is of the threshold needed for a positive response for any testing dilution that is the same or more concentrated/stronger than the glycerin control. For antigen dilutions that are equivalent or stronger than the glycerin control, a positive response is at least 7 mm and at least 2 mm larger than the wheal produced from the glycerin control. Tested antigen dilutions that are weaker than the glycerin control contain lower amounts of glycerin and the positive test criteria for those do not have to be altered.

Do you need a positive and negative control? Yes, because to make sure the skin reacts as expected. You need to confirm that it will react to histamine appropriately and that it won't react to things it shouldn't. See Chapter 14. You also need to know if there is glycerin sensitivity.

What's the positive control? The positive control is a diluted histamine solution prepared for intradermal testing. There are different concentrations of histamine made for different types of testing. Make sure to use the correct one. Generally, a diluted solution of aqueous histamine phosphate 0.275 mg/mL is used. Several preparation instructions are provided in this chapter.

What antigens to test? See Chapters 5 to 9. Try to tailor tests according to the patient. Include any relevant exposures. These tests are also used as part of protocols to test for medication allergies and venoms. Do not use these tests for food or chemical allergy testing.

Where to test the patient (in the office)? Same as skin testing—most commonly the volar surface of the forearm, arm, and back are used.

Could anaphylaxis really happen during intradermal testing? Yes! It's rare and unlikely, but patients may experience a variety of adverse events while testing. See Part 5, Allergy Emergencies, but the practitioner must be prepared to handle anaphylaxis if he/she chooses to do any form of skin testing.

16.3 Tools of the Trade (What Are Needed)

Short-beveled allergy testing syringes; larger syringes may be need for treatment board preparation (▶ Fig. 16.1a, b).
- Alcohol swabs or 70% isopropyl alcohol/gloves/skin marker/record sheet or electronic medical record (EMR) entry.
- Histamine prepared for intradermal skin testing.
- Negative control (PNS or some other liquid used as diluent); if needed, glycerin control(s).
- Testing/treatment board prepared with antigen dilutions (▶ Fig. 16.2).
- Emergency supplies (See Part 5, Allergy Emergencies)
- Wheal measuring device.

16.4 Shocking Information (How to Actually Do This!)

16.4.1 Preparation of Dilutions for the Testing/Treatment Board

Since various dilutions of antigens are used not just for patient testing, but also for immunotherapy, the procedure to make these dilutions are outlined in this section. Concentrated antigen is never used in intradermal testing. This procedure is also used to prepare histamine and glycerin controls.

To prepare the board, antigen concentrates are needed, syringes for mixing, and either 5-mL vials prefilled with 4 mL of PNS or 10-mL vials prefilled with 9 mL of PNS.

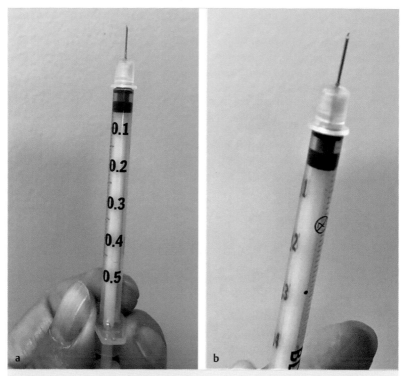

Fig. 16.1 (a) An example of an allergy testing syringe. Allergy testing and mixing syringes come as a single unit with a very small size syringe with attached needle. **(b)** An allergy testing syringe contains a short needle with short bevel.

All dilutions or immunotherapy vials (anything considered to be mixed or "compounded" for allergy testing and treatment purposes) must be prepared according to USP 797 guidelines, either under an ISO Class 5, primary engineering control (PEC) (▶ Fig. 16.3), OR in a dedicated allergenic extracts compounding area (AECA) by appropriately trained and regularly evaluated staff. See further details in Part 8.

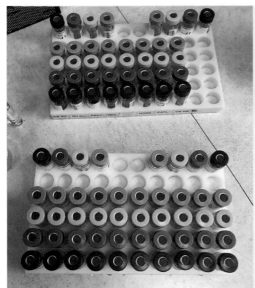

Fig. 16.2 An example of an allergy testing/treatment board. Displayed on the board are various antigens organized in rows by dilution and in columns by antigen. Note each color designated a certain dilution number. For example, the red-topped vials are all #1 dilutions of each antigen; the orange-topped vials are all #2 dilutions, etc.

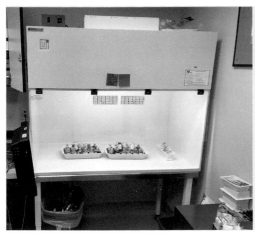

Fig. 16.3 An example of an allergy mixing area with an ISO Class 5, primary engineering control (PEC).

The dilutions used for testing and treatment are either 1:5 or 1:10 dilutions. If 1:5 dilutions is chosen, generally six different dilution strengths are prepared. If 1:10 dilutions are used, generally five dilution strengths are prepared. Before beginning the steps defined, ensure that mixing is done in an appropriate area and by personnel trained and evaluated according to USP 797 guidelines, all

needed equipment is ready, and the area (skin) to be tested is cleaned and prepared. Prepare labels for each dilution of each antigen prepared in advance.
Though preparation of these dilutions is monotonous and tedious, but it is
extremely important work, requiring careful attention to detail. It should be
performed in a quiet place, free of distractions.

Decide to use either 1:5 or 1:10, but not both. The dilution strengths are not
interchangeable so go with one or the other and stick with it. The author uses
1:5 dilutions those are discussed first.

Step 1

Clean tops of all vials to be used with alcohol swabs and allow them to dry
(▶ Fig. 16.4).

Step 2

Withdraw 1 mL of antigen concentrate and place it into either a 5-mL prefilled
vial to make a 1:5 dilution or a 10-mL prefilled vial to make a 1:10 dilution
(▶ Fig. 16.5a, b).

When injecting the antigen into the vial, do slowly to avoid foaming of the
solution.

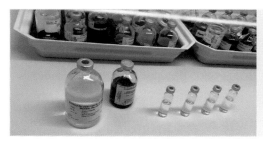

Fig. 16.4 An example of antigen concentrate, diluent, and
four 5-mL vials prefilled with
diluent prepared for making
1:5 dilutions.

Step 3

Gently mix the solution in the vial either by withdrawing and reinjecting a small amount of solution a few times or by agitating the vial gently (▶ Fig. 16.6).

Step 4

Label the vial for the particular antigen as Dilution #1 of that antigen.

Step 5

To make subsequent dilutions (#2–#5 or #6), repeat steps 2 to 4, but substitute the newly created dilution vial made in step 4 in place of the antigen concentrate vial (▶ Fig. 16.7 and ▶ Fig. 16.8).

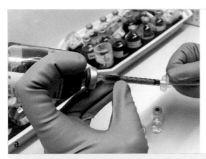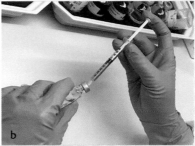

Fig. 16.5 (a) Withdraw 1 mL of antigen concentrate from the concentrate vial. **(b)** Inject the 1 mL of concentrate into the 5-mL vial prefilled with 4 mL of diluent to make a #1 dilution at a ratio of 1:5.

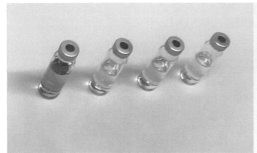

Fig. 16.6 The #1 dilution is ready to label. Notice the color change in the vial. Notice there is no foaming of antigen in the vial when mixed gently.

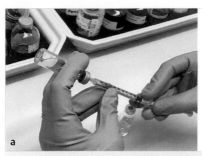
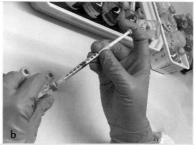

Fig. 16.7 **(a)** To make the #2 dilution, withdraw 1 mL from the #1 dilution vial. **(b)** Add the 1 mL from the #1 dilution vial to a new 5-mL vial prefilled with 4 mL of diluent to make a #2 dilution at a ratio of 1:5.

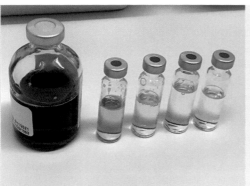

Fig. 16.8 Four completed dilutions are shown here (note the color change from the stronger dilution #1 to the weaker dilutions). Labels left off for demonstration purposes; be sure to always label yours.

Step 6

When all antigen dilution vials are prepared, be sure to organize them on the testing/treatment board and refrigerate them (see ▶ Fig. 16.2).

As an added safety measure in addition to clear labeling, it's helpful to color code the different dilutions. This can be done by purchasing prefilled vials with different colored tops or purchasing different colored caps that snap or close over the tops of the vials. Designate each dilution to be a different color (i.e., red is dilution #2).

16.4.2 Preparation of Controls

Histamine control: Aqueous histamine (not glycerinated) is used for intradermal testing. The strength is 0.275 mg/mL of histamine phosphate (0.1 mg/mL histamine base) and it is generally not used for intradermal testing straight from the vial. A histamine control can be prepared by using 1:5 dilutions to make a #3 dilution of histamine. See ▶ Table 16.1.

Glycerin control: For 1:5 dilutions, generally only intradermal tests using a #2 dilution require a glycerin control. A #2 dilution of antigen contains 2% glycerin; dilutions weaker than that generally do not have a strong enough glycerin concentration to irritate the skin. To make a glycerin control, use the 1:5 dilution technique to make a #2 glycerin dilution.

Negative (PNS) control: Requires no additional preparation. Use straight from the vial.

Table 16.1 Instructions for mixing a #3 histamine control for intradermal testing[a]

1. Obtain either three empty 5-mL vials or three unused 5-mL vials prefilled with 4 mL of PNS.

2. If using three empty vials, fill each vial with 4 mL of which diluent is being used (PNS, HSA).

3. Take 1 mL of the aqueous histamine phosphate 0.275 mg/mL and add it to one of the three 5-mL vials filled with 4 mL of diluent. Mix gently. Label as histamine dilution #1.

4. Take 1 mL of dilution #1 and add it to one of the three 5-mL vials filled with 4 mL of diluent. Mix gently. Label as histamine dilution #2.

5. Take 1 mL of dilution #2 and add it to one of the three 5-mL vials filled with 4 mL of diluent. Mix gently. Label as histamine dilution #3.

6. Keep and use histamine dilution #3. Discard dilutions #1 and #2.

Abbreviations: HSA, Human Serum Albumen; PNS, phenolated normal saline.
[a]These instructions assume the mixing area is prepped/cleaned, in an appropriate USP 797 approved space, and performed by trained personnel. This same technique is used to make glycerin controls.

16.4.3 Single Intradermal Testing Technique

Verify the following with the patient:
- Have they discontinued any interfering medications?
- Are they feeling well (not sick)?
- Have asthmatic patients suffered any recent exacerbations/rescue medication usage?
- Is the patient pregnant?

> If you have a spirometer in your clinic it is helpful to perform spirometry on suspected or known asthmatic patients prior to testing.

Step 1

Clean the area of skin being tested with an alcohol swab and allow area to dry.

Step 2

Withdraw a tiny amount (0.01–0.03 mL) of the chosen dilution to be injected into an allergy testing syringe with a short-beveled needle. Inject enough liquid to raise a 4-mm wheal.

Step 3

Using the nondominant hand, tense the skin and while keeping the syringe mostly parallel to the skin, insert the needle into the intradermal layer of the skin until the bevel disappears. Inject enough liquid to raise a 4-mm wheal. Measure the wheal to confirm it is 4 mm in size, unless you are highly skilled at this (► Fig. 16.9 and ► Fig. 16.10).

> To help with efficiency, especially when first starting out, press a 4-mm disposable otoscope speculum into the patient's skin. It will leave behind a 4-mm circular indentation in the skin that can be used as a helpful guide (► Fig. 16.11).
>
> This takes practice. If there's leakage of liquid, then the bevel wasn't completely covered by skin so the needle was not deep enough. If there's bleeding, the wheal edges are indistinct, or the wheal disappears before 10 minutes, the needle was placed too deep.

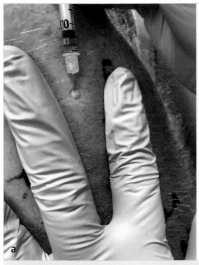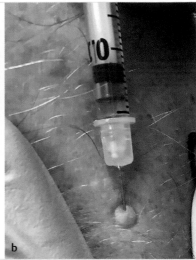

Fig. 16.9 (a) A single intradermal injection being pricked. The skin is tensed with the nondominant hand and the bevel is buried underneath the epidermis. Note the tiny volume of liquid within the syringe. **(b)** Close up of the intradermal injection. Note there is no bleeding.

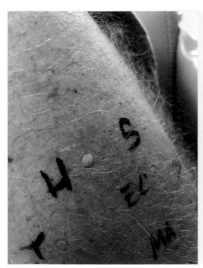

Fig. 16.10 A single intradermal skin test. Note there is no bleeding and the wheal is 4 mm in size.

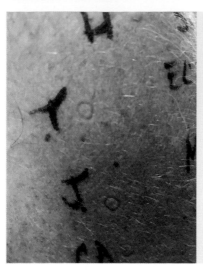

Fig. 16.11 An arm prepared for the first series of intradermal injections for intradermal dilutional testing by gently pressing a 4-mm disposable otoscope speculum into the skin to leave behind a series of 4 mm indentations.

Step 4

If applying multiple single intradermal tests, be sure to apply tests at least 2 cm apart from each other. This prevents false-positives from large spreading wheals.

Step 5

Once all tests are applied, wait for 10 minutes.

Step 6

Using a measuring device, measure each wheal and record it (▸ Fig. 16.12).

It is very helpful to palpate the wheal and tense the skin to make it easier to see for measurement.

Step 7

At this point, the patient should still have a pulse and respirations. Congratulations! The next challenge you face is to determine what you do with your test results. Good luck with that.

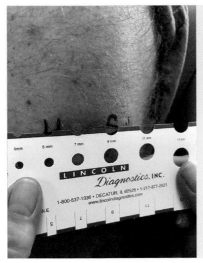

Fig. 16.12 After 10 minutes, the intradermal tests are read. Here is an example of a positive test (the histamine control) being read after 10 minutes. Note the size of the wheal.

16.4.4 Intradermal Dilutional Testing Technique

Intradermal dilutional testing (IDT) is a type of intradermal skin testing performed by some allergists to attempt to determine an "endpoint." An endpoint is a specific dilution that is thought to be a potential starting point for immunotherapy. It is generally performed using 1:5 dilutions, and usually involves placing dilutions in sequence from weakest to strongest starting with dilution #6 and proceeding, if applicable, to dilution #2. A #1 dilution is not placed, except in an attempt to "confirm" a #2 endpoint.

A dilution is considered to be the endpoint if it is the first positive wheal followed by a "confirmatory" wheal (▶ Fig. 16.13). A confirmatory wheal is a positive wheal that is 2 mm larger than the preceding positive wheal. In general, the first positive wheal usually turns out to be the endpoint. However, there are times when that first wheal is followed by another positive wheal which is not 2 mm larger. In the classic interpretation of IDT, an endpoint has not yet been reached and testing proceeds.

In the rare case where there are positive wheal responses, but no confirmatory wheal develops (called a "plateau response"), there is technically no endpoint determined in the classic interpretation of IDT. However, many providers will use the first positive wheal as the endpoint in this case.

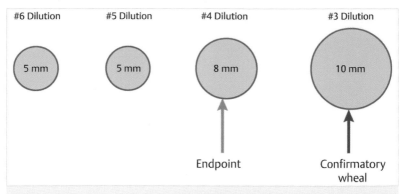

Fig. 16.13 An example of intradermal dilutional testing. In this example, the endpoint is dilution #4, because that is the first positive wheal followed by a confirmatory wheal—a wheal 2 mm larger than the preceding positive wheal.

When beginning to perform IDT, the #6 dilution is placed for all antigens being tested at one time. After waiting for 10 minutes and reading the results, #5 dilutions are placed of all tested antigens, then #4 dilutions, and so on. However, if a confirmatory wheal is found to validate an endpoint for a particular antigen, no further testing is done for that antigen (▶ Fig. 16.13). If all wheals of all dilutions placed are negative, then the test is negative for that antigen. Uncommonly, a "flash response" may occur. This is when a dilution is placed and the wheal grows markedly larger than the preceding wheal(s). While there is not a specific number in millimeters to define what is considered a flash response, if this happens, testing for that particular antigen should be stopped and performed another day (but the testing for other antigens may continue).

Once experienced with IDT, many practices will adapt the technique to save time. Some will start with #4 dilutions rather than #6 dilutions, some will place two or more dilutions at the same time (i.e., placing #6 and #5 dilutions for each antigen instead of just #6), and some will place every other dilution (#6, #4, #2). See ▶ Fig. 16.14 for an example of an adapted IDT set-up where #4 and #2 dilutions are used.

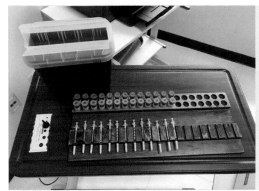

Fig. 16.14 An example of a set-up used for intradermal dilutional testing. In this case, #4 (pink vial tops) and #2 dilutions (orange vial tops) are mainly used.

Clinical Pearls **M!**

- Ensure that all dilutions, testing, and treatment vials are prepared according to USP 797 regulations by appropriately trained personnel in an appropriate area conforming to the regulations.
- Have testing supplies and the testing/treatment board prepared in advance of any testing.
- Dilutions (and immunotherapy treatment vials) should be prepared in a place free of distractions.
- Intradermal testing takes practice, be sure you and/or your nurses are doing it properly.
- Single intradermal testing can be used to diagnose allergic disease.
- IDT testing may help establish an endpoint to use as a guide for starting immunotherapy.
- Be prepared to handle anaphylaxis.

Bibliography

[1] King HC, Mabry RL, Gordon BR, et al. Allergy in ENT Practice: The Basic Guide. New York, NY: Thieme, 2004

[2] Wise SK, Lin SY, Toskala E, et al. International Consensus Statement on Allergy and Rhinology: Allergic Rhinitis. Int Forum Allergy Rhinol. 2018; 8(2):108–352

17 Skin Testing: Blended Techniques

Christine B. Franzese

17.1 Most Interesting Information

Skin prick testing is fast, reliable, and requires less skill to perform, but some allergists desire more information on the patient's level of sensitization or wish to determine an "endpoint" for an allergen, so this form of testing is inadequate for their needs. However, Intradermal Dilution Testing (IDT) is much more time-consuming, and requires more skill than skin prick testing. This is where blended testing techniques come in—the marriage of the speed with additional information, for those allergists who want it. The most well-known protocol is termed "modified quantitative testing (MQT)," and it involves combining the results of skin prick testing and single intradermal testing to determine an "endpoint," a potential starting point for immunotherapy.

17.2 Serious Stuff

Who's a good candidate for this type of skin testing? Anyone who's a candidate for skin prick and intradermal testing—patients with symptoms suggestive of immunoglobulin E (IgE)-mediated allergic disease and no medical contraindications listed in Chapters 15 and 16, and who have discontinued any interfering medications.

How does this test differ from skin prick testing or intradermal testing? What is the technique? The test is performed by placing a skin prick test for the antigens that are being tested. Then based on those results, a single intradermal test of two possible dilutions is placed. Based on the results of the skin prick and intradermal test, an endpoint can be assigned for each antigen tested. This technique has been discussed in more detail in this chapter.

What does this test tell? Similar to skin prick and intradermal, it shows whether or not IgE is present to (an) antigen(s). It can also be used to determine a starting point for immunotherapy, if that is desired.

What materials are needed? How are these tests performed? The materials used for prick and intradermal testing and the actual techniques to perform the prick and single intradermal tests are the same—see Chapters 16 and 17. The way in which the results of both are used is discussed further in this chapter.

How long does this test take? How do I read this test? The time is the same as discussed in Chapters 15 and 16 for both types of test: 20 minutes for prick testing, 10 minutes for intradermal testing. The criteria for positive and negative test interpretation are also the same—see Chapters 15 and 16.

What about controls? What controls are used? Do I have to place separate controls for each? The controls are the same as described in Chapter 15: A positive histamine control and negative 50% glycerin control for skin prick testing, and negative phenolated normal saline (PNS) and glycerin control for intradermal testing. However, it is not necessary to place two separate positive histamine tests, so the positive histamine control for intradermal testing can be skipped if the histamine control for prick testing responds appropriately.

What antigens to test for? See Chapters 5 to 9. The test should be tailored according to the patient. Any relevant exposures should be included. Do not use these tests for food or chemical allergy testing.

Where to test the patient (in the office)? Can the same area be used to test for both skin prick and intradermal? Again, most commonly the volar surface of the forearm, arm, and back are used. Whether it's a prick test or single intradermal test, each test needs to be 2 cm apart to prevent contamination and false-positives from large spreading wheals, so if the testing area can accommodate that then—Yes, that same area can be use. If not, the tests will need to be placed in separate areas; so plan accordingly.

Could anaphylaxis really happen during this type of testing? Yes! It's rare and unlikely, but patients may experience a variety of adverse events while testing. See Chapters 34 and 35, but the practitioner must be prepared to handle anaphylaxis while performing any form of skin testing.

17.3 Shocking Information (How to Actually Do This!)

17.3.1 Modified Quantitative Testing Protocol

In the previous chapters, the supplies needed for skin prick testing and intradermal testing, how to prepare dilutions and the controls needed, as well as the different testing techniques have been discussed. For clarification purposes, the dilutions used for intradermal testing are 1:5 dilutions, specifically the #2 and #5 dilution vials. As a reminder, an endpoint is a specific dilution that is thought to be a potential starting point for immunotherapy.

Verify the following with the patient:
• Have they discontinued any interfering medications?
• Are they feeling well (not sick)?
• Have asthmatic patients suffered any recent exacerbations/rescue medication usage?
• Is the patient pregnant?

If you have a spirometer in your clinic it is helpful to perform spirometry on suspected or known asthmatic patients prior to testing.

Step 1

Clean the area of skin being tested with an alcohol swab, allow area to dry, and make sure all the supplies are ready. Place the positive and negative controls needed for each type of test.

Step 2

Perform skin prick testing either with single or multi-prick devices for the selected antigens that are being tested.

Step 3

After 20 minutes, measure the wheal sizes and record them.

Step 4

For all antigens where the prick test is negative, place a #2 dilution single intradermal test. For all antigens where the prick test is positive, but the wheal size is less than 9 mm, place a #5 single intradermal test. For all antigens where the prick test is positive and the wheal was 9 mm or more in size, do nothing—these are considered to be a #6 endpoint and no further testing is required.

Step 5

Wait for 10 minutes, measure the wheal size, and record it.
  If the prick test is negative and:
- The #2 intradermal testing is negative, the antigen is negative.
- The #2 intradermal is positive; a #3 endpoint is assigned.

If the prick test is positive and:
- The #5 intradermal is negative; a #4 endpoint is assigned.
- The #5 intradermal is positive, but the wheal size is less than 9 mm in size, a #5 endpoint is assigned.
- The #5 intradermal is positive and the wheal size is 9 mm or greater, a #6 endpoint is assigned.

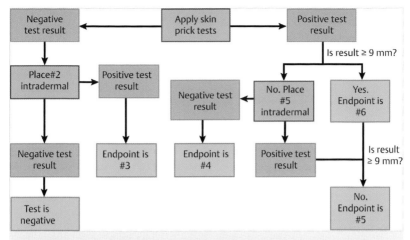

Fig. 17.1 Flowchart of the steps involved in modified quantitative testing (MQT) and results. Blue squares are action steps, orange squares are test results, and green squares are the final test determinations.

See ► Fig. 17.1 for a flowchart of this protocol.

Clinical Pearls   **M!**

- The materials and techniques to perform skin prick and single intradermal testing used in blended testing are the same—but the sequence of application and endpoint determination are different.
- If a skin prick testing wheal is 9 mm or greater, it's automatically #6 endpoint.
- Be prepared to handle anaphylaxis.

Bibliography

[1] King HC, Mabry RL, Gordon BR, et al. Allergy in ENT Practice: The Basic Guide. New York, NY: Thieme, 2004

[2] Wise SK, Lin SY, Toskala E, et al. International Consensus Statement on Allergy and Rhinology: Allergic Rhinitis. Int Forum Allergy Rhinol. 2018; 8(2):108–352

18 Specific Immunoglobulin E Testing for Inhalant Allergy

James W. Mims, Matthew W. Ryan, Cecelia C. Damask

18.1 Getting Serious About Serum

When a patient is allergic to birch pollen, exposure to birch pollen causes mast cells to degranulate, releasing allergic mediators such as histamine. Immunoglobulin E (IgE) is the molecule on the surface of the mast cell that binds to part of the birch pollen. IgE is not produced by mast cells, it is produced by plasma cells and travels to bind to IgE receptors found on different inflammatory cell types including mast cells, basophils, eosinophils, and lymphocytes. When attached to a mast cell or basophil, degranulation is signaled when two molecules of specific IgE (sIgE) both bind (or cross-link) to the allergen. The role of IgE receptors on other inflammatory cells (such as antigen presenting cells and lymphocytes) is less clear but assumed to be involved with the regulation of allergic inflammation. As IgE produced by plasma cells travels through the circulation to IgE receptors in tissue, IgE can be sampled from sera or plasma. Even with this simplified explanation of the allergic immune process, it is easy to speculate that many factors would affect the presence or magnitude of the allergic reaction (such as the number, stability, and location of mast cells, the quantity of histamine in the mast cell granules, the expression of histamine receptors, etc.). However, the presence of sIgE would be a necessary component of an IgE-mediated allergy by definition.

The technique for measuring sIgE has not changed conceptually since 1967, although the particulars of the technique have been refined, which has substantially improved the sensitivity and specificity of the testing. The sensitivity and specificity for sIgE testing has been primarily compared to skin testing because of the historic role skin testing has held in allergy evaluation.

18.2 Technique for Measuring sIgE

Blood collected from the test subject is centrifuged and the serum is separated. (Plasma and sera show essentially the same results.) The serum is analyzed for sIgE. Conceptually, a series of five steps is common to all sIgE testing. This process has been illustrated using cat allergy as an example.

18.2.1 Step 1: Incubation

Particles containing cat allergen (e.g., cat dander) are bound to a matrix, such as a string, paper, bead, or sponge, so that the allergen does not wash away

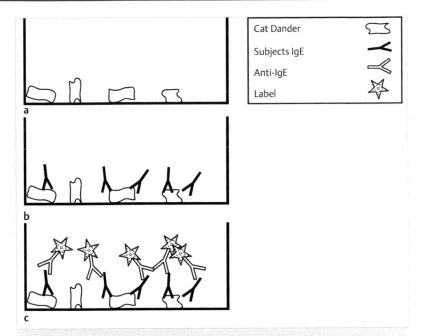

Fig. 18.1 (a) Allergen particles (example: cat dander) are bound to a matrix. **(b)** The subject's plasma or sera is added and cat dander-specific immunoglobulin will bind. The remaining sera is rinsed away. **(c)** A labeled anti-IgE IgG is used to tag the bound IgE. The label (star) may then be measured. IgE, immunoglobulin E; IgG, immunoglobulin G.

during the testing. One could imagine cat dander glued to the sides of a test tube (▸ Fig. 18.1a). Serum from the subject is then exposed to the matrix with the affixed cat allergen for a set period of time. Only the IgE specific to cat allergens should bind to the cat dander (▸ Fig. 18.1b).

18.2.2 Step 2: First rinse

The serum is rinsed away after the cat specific IgE has had time to bind. This washing process is done to remove all the other IgE that is not bound to the cat dander.

18.2.3 Step 3: Labeling

The subject's cat-specific IgE that is bound to the cat allergen is tagged using a labeled anti-IgE antibody. Anti-human IgE antibody is formed when the serum from another species of animal (such as a rabbit) is injected with human IgE.

The rabbit produces IgG against the human IgE. In the lab, different markers can be attached to the fragment crystallizable region (Fc region) of the rabbit IgG. During sIgE testing, labeled rabbit anti-IgE immunoglobulin will bind to the sIgE, which is bound to the cat allergen fixed to a matrix (► Fig. 18.1c).

18.2.4 Step 4: Second rinse

Wash away the excess (unbound) anti-IgE rabbit immunoglobulin.

18.2.5 Step 5: Measurement

Measure and quantify how much labeled anti-IgE remains bound to the cat-specific IgE (which is bound to the fixed cat antigen).

In practice, each step presents technical issues. Isolating the allergen from biologic sources has all the standardization problems as creating allergen extracts. As in skin testing, sIgE testing is only as good as the source and processing of the allergen. Binding the allergen to the matrix without disrupting its antigenicity can be problematic. Washing away the unbound IgE (which likes to stick to the sidewalls) without disrupting the bound IgE or bound allergen is critical. The anti-IgE is biologically produced but needs to be consistent in its binding to the IgE. And the labeling is difficult because there is not much sIgE in the sera, so the label has to be amplified while providing consistent results.

The history of sIgE testing has led to multiple different names in the literature. Specific IgE testing is sometimes called "in vitro" allergy testing as it is performed outside of the body. Brand names of sIgE test systems such as ImmunoCap, Hytec, and Immulite are sometimes used. Other studies refer to elevated sIgE as seroatopy, and many clinicians still say "RAST" (and modified RAST is still commercially available).

18.3 Comparisons Between IgE Testing and Skin Testing

The advantages of skin testing and sIgE testing are summarized in ► Table 18.1 and ► Table 18.2. There is no simple answer as to which is the best inhalant allergen test. However, knowing how the tests compare is useful for interpreting sIgE test results.

Table 18.1 Advantages of sIgE testing compared to skin testing

No local or systemic reactions

Single venipuncture

Not affected my medications (such as antihistamines)

Quantitative information (compared to skin prick test alone)

Not affected by skin conditions (dermatographia)

sIge/tIgE ratio may be useful

Skin test results involve subjective comparison to controls

Future benefit of component testing

Abbreviations: sIgE, specific immunoglobulin E; tIgE, total immunoglobulin E.

Table 18.2 Advantages of skin testing compared to sIgE testing

Results visible to patient

Results available in minutes

Prick tests easier to apply than venipuncture

Skin prick tests likely more sensitive than sIgE testing

Skin prick tests less expensive per test

Same allergen extract can be used for testing and immunotherapy

Abbreviation: sIgE, specific immunoglobulin E.

18.4 Sensitivity and Specificity

The comparison of sIgE testing and skin testing inherently varies with the allergen tested, the criteria for determining the skin test as positive, and the true frequency of allergic disease in the population tested. As such, a global statement would be inappropriate.

As a positive skin prick test can be seen in the absence of clinical disease, it is unclear which test most accurately predicts clinical disease. Studies evaluating skin test positive and sIgE-negative subjects by seasonal symptom records or challenge tests have not been performed. It would also be interesting to know if skin prick test positive but sIgE-negative patients would benefit from immunotherapy in a placebo-controlled trial. It would be difficult to recruit enough subjects for this study.

18.5 Other Advantages and Disadvantages

Specific IgE testing should have the same risks as a routine blood collected with no risk of an allergic reaction. While there is a potential safety advantage to sIgE testing over prick testing, the practical benefit is very small. Skin testing has the convenience of providing results within minutes. Specific IgE testing has the convenience of a single needle stick, no skin reactions, not being affected by skin conditions (dermatographia), and not being affected by medications (such as antihistamines). When considering immunotherapy, skin testing has the advantage that the same extract can be used for testing and treatment. Immunotherapy based on sIgE requires a change of manufacturer between testing and treatment. The difference between the manufactures' allergen procurement is subject to biological variability especially in nonstandardized extracts. This may lead the practitioner to start immunotherapy at a lower dose which would prolong the escalation phase of immunotherapy. Quantification provided by sIgE testing may allow immunotherapy to be started at higher doses compared to skin prick test alone. However, this benefit would be lost if most immunotherapy patients had high levels of sIgE.

18.6 Interpretation of sIgE Testing

The diagnosis of allergy is not a straightforward process. Clinicians are faced with three dilemmas. First, allergy testing can be positive in individuals without significant clinical manifestations. Second, clinical manifestations of allergic rhinitis overlap with symptoms of nonallergic rhinitis and chronic rhinosinusitis. Inflammatory responses to irritants, such as tobacco smoke, bacteria, and viruses further complicate the diagnostic issue. Third, negative allergy testing does not eliminate allergy from the differential diagnosis (but makes it less likely).

Specific IgE and total IgE (tIgE) can be reported in three ways according to national laboratory guidelines: (1) qualitative (positive/negative), (2) semi-quantitative (arbitrary units kU/L), or (3) quantitative (referenced to WHO 75/502 in mg/L or kU_A/L). The techniques used currently generally report single sIgE test and tIgE test quantitatively, and combination allergen "screens" as qualitative. Quantitative sIgE results are divided into classes (▶ Table 18.3) by most manufacturers. (Classes were initially derived from dilutions of pooled sera from highly birch-allergic subjects.) Despite quantitative reporting, significant variation can exist between different technologies as the source allergens used in the testing is not uniformly standardized. Despite these problems, quantification of the sIgE has clinical utility.

Table 18.3 sIgE semi-quantitative classes

Quantitative results (kUA/l)	Level of allergen-specific antibody	Semi-quantitative results (specific IgE class)
<0.35	Absent or undetectable	0
0.35 to<0.7	Low	1
0.7 to<3.5	Moderate	2
3.5 to<17.5	High	3
17.5 to<50	Very high	4
50 to<100	Very high	5
100 and larger	Very high	6

While symptom severity has not been shown to correlate well with skin test reactivity or sIgE levels, research supports the principle that as IgE levels increase the probability of clinical symptoms also increases. This has led to the notion that certain levels of sIgE can achieve a 95% confidence that the allergen causes symptoms. Hugh Sampson demonstrated this clearly in peanut allergy by comparing the likelihood of a positive double-blind placebo-controlled food challenge with the sIgE level for peanut. He showed that if the sIgE for peanut is more than 15 kU_A/L then there is more than 95% chance of a positive response after a placebo-controlled food challenge. Similar findings were shown for inhalant allergens by Pastorello et al in 1995 and Ahlstedt in 2002. Unfortunately, the probability curves would be expected to shift by allergen, technology, and criteria for "clinical allergy" of the subjects tested. Nevertheless, high levels of a sIgE are more likely associated with the patient having clinical symptoms than low levels are. The clinician should balance their clinical impression with the test results to determine if the allergen exposure is playing a role.

18.7 Future of sIgE Testing

18.7.1 "Component" Testing

IgE recognizes small series of amino acids (epitopes) on proteins or glycoproteins. An allergen source frequently has multiple proteins contributing to the allergenicity and there may be more than one epitope recognized per protein. The proteins travel on particles such as dust mite feces or cat dander. Allergy extracts used for skin and sIgE testing tend to contain the particles associated with the antigen source. The allergic proteins are named by a convention using the first three letters of the genus, the first letter of the species, and sequential numbers as allergens are discovered. The first cat (*Felis domesticus*) allergen discovered is named Fel d 1. Component testing involves placing the different proteins or epitopes on a microchip and measuring the IgE to each component of the source independently.

Component testing for peanut allergy is now commercially approved in the United States. Studies on peanut and latex suggest that component testing may give us insight as to which components are associated with clinical manifestations. In peanut, Ara H1, 2, and sometimes 3 are associated with clinical manifestations, and multicomponent sensitization is associated with severity. Additionally, some peanut components, such as Ara H8 are cross-reactive with birch. Component testing may be able to demonstrate false-positive whole peanut test results and differentiate "mild" peanut allergy such as oral allergy syndrome, from cases at risk for anaphylaxis. In latex, Hev b 1, 3, 5, 6 may be more important than Hev b 8 in causing clinical manifestations. The field of component testing is new, but will certainly become more important over time. The expanded use of component testing will depend upon additional data that demonstrate the clinical significance of sIgE against particular components as well as payer policies regarding coverage. Immunotherapy is still performed with crude extracts, and until specific component immunotherapy is available, the role of component testing will be confined to prognostication and delineation of cross-reactivity.

Clinical Pearls   M!

- Positive allergy skin tests and specific IgE (sIgE) tests are more common than clinical allergy and are not equivalent with clinical allergic disease.
- There is no "gold standard" for testing inhalant allergens. Skin testing and sIgE testing offer different advantages in evaluating the potentially allergic patient.
- Studies differ regarding the relative sensitivity and specificity of sIgE compared to skin testing. Skin prick testing may be more sensitive for some allergens.
- Specific IgE testing is quantified against a standard set by the World Health Organization. In the United States sIgE testing is subject to national laboratory standards as regulated by the Clinical Laboratory Improvement Amendments (CLIA).

Bibliography

[1] Bernstein IL, Li JT, Bernstein DI, et al. American Academy of Allergy, Asthma and Immunology, American College of Allergy, Asthma and Immunology. Allergy diagnostic testing: an updated practice parameter. Ann Allergy Asthma Immunol. 2008; 100(3) Suppl 3:S1–S148

[2] Moyer DB, Nelson HS. Use of modified radioallergosorbent testing in determining initial immunotherapy doses. Otolaryngol Head Neck Surg. 1985; 93(3):335–338

[3] Nam YH, Lee SK. Comparison between skin prick test and serum immunoglobulin E by CAP system to inhalant allergens. Ann Allergy Asthma Immunol. 2017; 118(5):608–613

[4] Plebani M. Clinical value and measurement of specific IgE. Clin Biochem. 2003; 36(6):453–469

19 Environmental Avoidance

Sarah K. Wise

19.1 A Word About Avoidance

In the traditional three-pronged treatment approach for allergic conditions, allergen avoidance (or environmental control [EC]) is often advocated. The remaining two arms of classic treatment for allergy are pharmacotherapy and allergen immunotherapy. Patients are frequently very interested in being educated on allergen avoidance and EC. Interestingly, however, the evidence for the efficacy of these measures is weaker than the evidence for many pharmacotherapy and allergen immunotherapy modalities, especially with respect to respiratory symptom outcomes. This chapter will examine environmental avoidance measures for dust mite, pet dander, cockroach, and pollen allergens, as well as the evidence for their efficacy.

19.2 Serious Stuff

19.2.1 Do Dust Mite Environmental Control Measures Work?

House dust mites (HDM), most commonly *Dermatophagoides farinae* in the United States and *Dermatophagoides pteronyssinus* in Europe, are common perennial allergens. EC measures for HDM may include physical methods and chemical treatments. Physical modalities include heating, freezing, barrier methods, air filtration and ventilation, vacuuming, and others. The efficacy of these physical techniques has been studied for the treatment of HDM-allergic rhinitis (AR). Findings across studies are varied. Most commonly, HDM antigen levels are decreased in the environment in which the physical techniques are used. However, improvement in respiratory symptoms has not been reliably confirmed. Studies investigating clinical improvement with HDM-impermeable bedding or high efficiency particulate air (HEPA) filtration generally failed to show clinical benefit.

Acaricides are chemical treatments to decrease HDM concentration. The use of acaricides has been shown to improve symptoms in allergic patients with HDM sensitization. No serious adverse effects were reported from these interventions.

In 2010, a Cochrane review evaluated EC measures for HDM-AR, including impermeable covers, HEPA filters, acaricides, or combination treatments. The authors of this systematic review noted significant methodological limitations in the studies that examined EC measures for HDM control in the perennial AR patients. Nonetheless, of all interventions, they noted that acaricides appeared to be the most promising and HDM impermeable bedding alone was unlikely to provide benefit. Overall, EC measures to treat AR with HDM sensitivity are considered an option.

19.2.2 Little Johnny Has a Cat Allergy. He Has to Get Rid of Fluffy the Cat. Right?

Pet removal is commonly advocated in the treatment strategy for AR patients with pet sensitivity. However, high-quality outcome studies are generally lacking for this intervention. In addition, compliance rates for pet removal are low.

Several studies have assessed EC for pet-sensitive allergic patients and their results are mixed. For multimodality EC measures, significant improvements in clinical symptoms and nasal airflow have been demonstrated. However, single-modality EC interventions generally do not result in improved symptoms, even if antigen levels are reduced. Studies of single-modality interventions have included HEPA filtration and pet washing. Furthermore, washing pets (cat and dog) must be performed twice a week in order to keep antigen levels low, and with removal of pets it may take several months to reduce antigen levels. Of note, current asthma treatment guidelines recommend removal of pets from a sensitized patient's home, as asthma may be secondarily prevented when sensitized patients avoid pets. Current aggregate evidence for pet avoidance and EC measures is level B, with an option to incorporate this treatment for the AR patient with pet sensitivity.

19.2.3 Cockroaches. Disgusting! Can We Control Cockroaches to Alleviate Allergic Symptoms?

Cockroaches are common in inner city areas but may also be present in rural homes in warm climates. EC measures for cockroach are aimed at decreasing the level of cockroach allergen and/or eliminating cockroach manifestations. There are three primary strategies for controlling cockroach allergen in the home: (1) education-based methods [e.g. instruction on house cleaning measures and sealing cracks/crevices]; (2) physical methods using insecticides or bait traps; and (3) combination therapy with both education-based interventions and physical methods.

Studies conducted for cockroach EC have shown that professional pest control is the most effective treatment for eliminating infestation and reducing allergen load. Bait traps appear to be more effective than insecticides placed on baseboards, cracks, and crevices. In addition, bait traps (including labor and monitoring costs) are less expensive than insecticide application. Of note, adherence to home-based EC measures for cockroach elimination is relatively poor.

While there have been several controlled trials assessing the efficacy of EC measures to eliminate cockroaches or reduce the levels of Bla g 1 and Bla g 2, outcomes related to respiratory symptoms or respiratory health are not routinely reported. In fact, in a recent review, it was noted that no studies included any assessment of symptoms associated with AR or its treatment. Furthermore, despite a reduction in allergen in studies implementing EC measures for cockroach, often the residual levels of allergen remained higher than median acceptable levels, and reinfestation is a continued concern in multi-family dwellings. EC measures for cockroach are considered an option, with aggregate grade of evidence B.

19.2.4 It's Spring Time and the Pollen Is Everywhere. There's No Way to Control This, Is There?

To decrease allergen exposure during the respective pollen season, EC measures for pollen allergy are used. However, it is practically impossible to completely avoid pollen exposure as outdoor pollination occurs naturally. Although there are some common techniques to decrease patients' exposure to pollen by avoidance measures, few clinical studies evaluate the efficacy of these interventions.

Patients may obtain information about the pollen count through online or media outlets. When the outdoor pollen count is high, a patient who is sensitive may choose to decrease outdoor exposure and/or adjust targeted medication. Expert opinion supports these techniques, but there is essentially no evidence in support of their efficacy. Other interventions such as closing windows during high pollen counts, specialized pollen filters in the car, removal of pollen-exposed clothing, and washing hair before bed have been advocated by experts. Similarly, there are no clinical studies to support these interventions.

A specific physical barrier method, wraparound eye glasses, has been studied in a controlled trial and found to be effective for nasal and ocular symptom control in seasonal AR patients. Another physical method, use of an active nasal filter that removes particles from inhaled air, has also been studied in a double-blind randomized controlled trial and found to be effective for nasal symptom control.

Considering the sum of the available evidence, EC measures for pollen allergy have an aggregate grade of evidence of B and are considered an option for the treatment of the AR patient.

> **Clinical Pearls** **M!**
>
> - While allergic patients are very keen to learn about EC measures, the evidence for their efficacy in controlling AR symptoms is somewhat weaker than for other treatment measures.
> - In general, EC measures carry an aggregate level of evidence B and are considered an option for the treatment of AR.
> - The strongest evidence for allergen avoidance measures demonstrating symptom benefit lies with dust mite ECs. The use of acaricides has shown to be the most beneficial of any single measure, although multimodality ECs are typically advocated.

Bibliography

[1] Comert S, Karakaya G, Kalyoncu AF. Wraparound eyeglasses improve symptoms and quality of life in patients with seasonal allergic rhinoconjunctivitis. Int Forum Allergy Rhinol. 2016; 6(7): 722–730

[2] Kenney P, Hilberg O, Pedersen H, Nielsen OB, Sigsgaard T. Nasal filters for the treatment of allergic rhinitis: a randomized, double-blind, placebo-controlled crossover clinical trial. J Allergy Clin Immunol. 2014; 133(5):1477–1480, 1480.e1–1480.e13

[3] Le Cann P, Paulus H, Glorennec P, Le Bot B, Frain S, Gangneux JP. Home environmental interventions for the prevention or control of allergic and respiratory diseases: what really works. J Allergy Clin Immunol Pract. 2017; 5(1):66–79

[4] Nurmatov U, van Schayck CP, Hurwitz B, Sheikh A. House dust mite avoidance measures for perennial allergic rhinitis: an updated Cochrane systematic review. Allergy. 2012; 67(2):158–165

[5] Wise SK, Lin SY, Toskala E, et al. International Consensus Statement on Allergy and Rhinology: Allergic Rhinitis. Int Forum Allergy Rhinol. 2018; 8(2):108–352

20 Pharmacotherapy: Decongestants

Christine B. Franzese

20.1 A Word of Caution

This section of the book contains information on the various medication options available to treat allergy symptoms. In each chapter, you'll find high-yield information on what each class of medication is, what symptoms each class is good in treating, examples of the class, why/when you might choose to use each either alone or in combination, and associated risks/side effects.

For this chapter, the author's take-home point is: Beware! Although decongestants are frequently used to treat allergic symptoms, these medications are not specifically focused on targeting allergies and the author avoids using these. They are generally not meant for long-term daily use and have significant side effects and risks. There are few select times when the author has recommended their use to patients. However, the practitioner should use them with caution for treating allergy symptoms, particularly for any extended period of time.

20.2 What Is This Class of Medication?

These medications act on alpha adrenergic receptors and one of their main effects is vasoconstriction. Intranasal decongestants also thin the nasal mucosa.

20.3 What Symptoms Are Good for Treating?

Nasal congestion, ocular erythema. These medications cause vasoconstriction, which shrinks blood vessels, reducing nasal congestion symptoms and the appearance of red eyes. However, they have no effect on other allergy symptoms, such as sneezing, rhinorrhea, or itchiness.

20.4 Examples of This Class

Intranasal decongestants: Oxymetazoline, xylometazoline, phenylephrine (6 years of age and older, unless physician-recommended)
Ocular decongestants: Phenylephrine 0.12%, tetrahydrozoline 0.05%, naphazoline 0.12% (6 years of age and older, unless physician-recommended)
Oral decongestants: Pseudoephedrine, phenylephrine (6 years of age and older)

Pseudoephedrine has been shown to be more effective in relieving intranasal symptoms than phenylephrine.

20.5 Why and When to Use

Rarely. Only when symptoms are severe and/or to help improve the delivery of other therapies, such as intranasal topical corticosteroids or saline rinses/sprays. Consider brief use restricted to 3 to 5 days at most. This recommendation for rare or brief use includes the combination antihistamine–decongestant combinations.

20.6 Risks and Side Effects

Oral decongestants: Insomnia, nervousness, anxiety, tremors, heart palpitations, increased blood pressure (both systolic and diastolic)

Use with caution in patients at risk for high blood pressure, who have hypertension, or are at risk for associated complications of hypertension (heart attack, stroke, etc.

Intranasal decongestants: Stinging, burning, dryness, nasal mucosal ulcerations, epistaxis

Rhinitis medicamentosa: The condition where prolonged use of intranasal antihistamines leads to medication tolerance and rebound congestion. While the exact dosage and duration that leads to rhinitis medicamentosa is unknown, it is best to stick with short courses of these medications.

Ocular decongestants: Rebound ocular erythema, pupillary dilation; contraindicated in narrow-angle glaucoma

Chronic use can possibly lead to toxic follicular reactions and contact dermatitis.

20.7 A Special Word on Antihistamine–Decongestant Combinations (Oral, Ocular Preparations)

Consider avoiding routine use of the antihistamine–decongestant combinations. While adding an oral decongestant to an antihistamine helps improve nasal congestion symptoms, the added risks of this class of medication outweigh the benefits of symptom improvement due to the fact that antihistamine–decongestant combinations are marketed for daily use and many patients continue taking these combination medications for long term without monitoring their blood pressure or being aware of the risks of long-term use.

⚠

Antihistamines have no effect on nasal congestion.

Clinical Pearls

- These medications are for short-term use; avoid long-term use.
- Make patients aware of potential side effects when using these medications.

Bibliography

[1] Horak F, Zieglmayer P, Zieglmayer R, et al. A placebo-controlled study of the nasal decongestant effect of phenylephrine and pseudoephedrine in the Vienna Challenge Chamber. Ann Allergy Asthma Immunol. 2009; 102(2):116–120

[2] Salerno SM, Jackson JL, Berbano EP. Effect of oral pseudoephedrine on blood pressure and heart rate: a meta-analysis. Arch Intern Med. 2005; 165(15):1686–1694

[3] Soparkar CN, Wilhelmus KR, Koch DD, Wallace GW, Jones DB. Acute and chronic conjunctivitis due to over-the-counter ophthalmic decongestants. Arch Ophthalmol. 1997; 115(1):34–38

[4] Wise SK, Lin SY, Toskala E, et al. International Consensus Statement on Allergy and Rhinology: Allergic Rhinitis. Int Forum Allergy Rhinol. 2018; 8(2):108–352

21 Anticholinergics

Christine B. Franzese

21.1 When the Nose Runs Like a Faucet

This chapter deals exclusively with anticholinergic nasal sprays. While there are metered-dose inhaler and nebulized versions of this medication, the formulations and their uses are not considered here. Anticholinergic nasal sprays are particularly useful for watery rhinorrhea, particularly in older people who complain of this type of symptom.

21.2 What Is This Class of Medication?

Anticholinergic medications act on the parasympathetic nervous system and block the binding of acetylcholine to muscarinic receptors on mucus glands. Simulation of parasympathetic fibers activates mucus glands to produce a watery discharge. This class blocks that activation.

21.3 What Symptoms Are Good for Treating?

These medications are good for treating watery rhinorrhea. These medicines are extremely good at drying up the nose. It is very useful in treating senile rhinitis, gustatory rhinitis, vasomotor rhinitis, rhinitis secondary to viral infections, among other things. It can be used to treat rhinorrhea associated with allergies, but has little to no effect on other allergic symptoms, such as sneezing and congestion.

21.4 Examples of This Class

Intranasal: Ipratropium bromide 0.03%, 0.06% (6 years and older)

21.5 Why and When to Use

These medications are used for treating complaints of watery nasal drainage or profuse clear rhinorrhea; more useful in nonallergic types of rhinitis given its lack of effectiveness on sneezing and nasal congestion.

It is fast acting and of short duration, may be used 4 to 6 times a day.

These medications can be combined with intranasal steroid use. The combination of intranasal and anticholinergic nasal sprays has been found to be more effective than either agent alone in treating rhinorrhea. Consider adding this agent in patients on intranasal steroids with an incomplete response and complaints of continued rhinorrhea.

21.6 Risks and Side Effects

Local: Nasal dryness and crusting, epistaxis, nasal irritation
Systemic: (Rare) dry mouth, dry/irritated eyes, blurred vision

Clinical Pearls   M!

- Useful in senile rhinitis, viral rhinitis, gustatory rhinitis, and other nonallergic types of rhinitis.

Bibliography

[1] Kim KT, Kerwin E, Landwehr L, et al. Pediatric Atrovent Nasal Spray Study Group. Use of 0.06% ipratropium bromide nasal spray in children aged 2 to 5 years with rhinorrhea due to a common cold or allergies. Ann Allergy Asthma Immunol. 2005; 94(1):73–79

[2] Naclerio R. Anticholinergic drugs in nonallergic rhinitis. World Allergy Organ J. 2009; 2(8): 162–165

22 Antihistamines

Christine B. Franzese

22.1 One of the Workhorses of Allergy Medications

Antihistamines are the major workhorse medications in the treatment of allergic disorders. This chapter will review oral H1 and H2 antihistamines, as well as intranasal and ocular antihistamines.

22.2 What Is This Class of Medication?

Histamine is one of the primary mediators of the allergic cascade and responsible for symptoms of sneezing, itching, nasal congestion, and rhinorrhea, among others. Histamine release is what generates the wheal and flare reaction seen in skin testing. Antihistamines work by blocking the binding of histamine to receptors. H1 antihistamines block binding to H1 receptors, and H2 antihistamines block binding to H2 receptors.

H1 antihistamines are further divided into first-generation and later-generation antihistamines. The first-generation H1 blockers cross the blood-brain barrier to a greater degree than later-generation H1 blockers. This leads to more frequent cognitive side effects, as well as some anticholinergic side effects, such as dry mouth. They also act as inhibitors of some liver enzymes, such as CYP2D6, which may cause them to effect the metabolism of other drugs. For this reason, first-generation antihistamines are not recommended for the treatment of allergic rhinitis.

H2 antihistamines have a larger impact on gastric acid secretion than on allergic symptoms and their usefulness in treating allergic rhinitis has not been definitively proven. However, they may impact skin testing and occasionally, some practitioners will use H1 and H2 antihistamines in combination to treat allergic rhinitis.

22.3 What Symptoms Are Good for Treating?

Oral H1 antihistamines (all generations): Sneezing, itching, rhinorrhea, and hives; can be used for ocular itching, redness, and tearing, but intranasal antihistamines have a better effect on these symptoms.

No oral antihistamine has any effect on nasal congestion.

Oral H2 antihistamines: Clinical benefit in allergic rhinitis is unclear.

Intranasal antihistamines: Nasal congestion, sneezing, nasal itching, rhinorrhea, eye symptoms (itching, redness, conjunctival edema, tearing). These sprays have a rapid onset of action (as quickly as 15 minutes).

Ocular antihistamines: Eye itching, redness, and conjunctival edema.

22.4 Examples of This Class

Oral H1 antihistamines (first generation): Diphenhydramine, chlorpheniramine, brompheniramine

Oral H1 antihistamines (later generations): Fexofenadine, loratadine, cetirizine, desloratadine, levocetirizine

Oral H2 antihistamines: Ranitidine, famotidine

Intranasal antihistamines: Azelastine (0.1%, 0.15%) and olopatadine

Ocular antihistamines: Azelastine, epinastine, emedastine, cetirizine, alcaftadine

22.5 Why and When to Use

Oral H1 antihistamines (first generation): Avoid routine use for typical symptoms of allergic rhinitis. Consider short-term use when symptoms are severe or for acute treatment of allergic reactions.

Oral H1 antihistamines (later generation): Use when the primary symptoms are sneezing, itching, hives, rhinorrhea, mild nasal obstruction symptoms. These may help with eye symptoms. Avoid for primary symptoms of nasal congestion, where an intranasal antihistamine or intranasal steroid spray would be more effective.

Oral H2 antihistamines: Not useful alone to treat allergic symptoms. Some may be used in combination with H1 blockers.

Intranasal antihistamines: Useful for symptoms of nasal congestion, sneezing, rhinorrhea, and nasal itching. Some studies have shown that these are more effective for eye and nasal symptoms than intranasal steroids, and more effective on nasal symptoms than oral H1 antihistamines. Due to the fast onset of action, these can be very useful in treating patients that like the effects of intranasal or oral decongestants.

They can also be helpful in rhinitis medicamentosa to wean patients off intranasal decongestants.

Ocular antihistamines: Useful for isolated allergic eye symptoms; also useful in eye symptoms resistant to other classes of allergy medications.

22.6 Risks and Side Effects

Oral H1 antihistamines (first generation): Drowsiness and sedation, impaired concentration, dizziness, fatigue, difficulty with memory, dry mouth

These medications can affect the metabolism of β blockers, anti-arrhythmics, tricyclic antidepressants, among others. This is another reason to avoid their use, especially in older patients.

Oral H1 antihistamines (later generations): Sedation, headache, fatigue, dry mouth, dizziness
Oral H2 antihistamines: Headache, dizziness, diarrhea, constipation
Intranasal antihistamines: Bitter taste, sedation, headache, epistaxis
Ocular antihistamines: Headache, blurred vision, burning, stinging, dry eye

22.7 Ages for Use

Oral H1 antihistamines (first generation): Varies widely. Some oral H1 antihistamines are not recommended to use in children below the age 4 to 6 years.
Oral H1 antihistamines (later generations): Levocetirizine and desloratadine can be used in children from age 6 months onward; cetirizine, loratadine, and fexofenadine can be used in children from age 2 onward.
Oral H2 antihistamines: Ranitidine and famotidine can be used in children from age 1 month onward.
Intranasal antihistamines: Azelastine and olopatadine can be used in children from age 5–6 years onward.

Astepro (brand of Azelastine 0.1%) is approved for perennial allergic rhinitis symptoms down to 6 months of age.

Ocular antihistamines: Alcaftadine, epinastine, and cetirizine can be used in children from age 2 onward; azelastine and emedastine can be used in children from age 3 onward.

Clinical Pearls   M!

- Antihistamines are good for treating symptoms of allergic rhinitis except for congestion.
- Avoid if patient's primary complaint is congestion, unless prescribing an intranasal antihistamine.
- Be sure to aware patients about side effects, such as sedation.
- Although eye symptoms will sometimes respond to oral antihistamines, many times a separate eye drop is prescribed depending on syptoms.

Bibliography

[1] Brozek JL, Bousquet J, Baena-Cagnani CE, et al. Global Allergy and Asthma European Network, Grading of Recommendations Assessment, Development and Evaluation Working Group. Allergic Rhinitis and its Impact on Asthma (ARIA) guidelines: 2010 revision. J Allergy Clin Immunol. 2010; 126(3):466–476

[2] Taylor-Clark T, Sodha R, Warner B, Foreman J. Histamine receptors that influence blockage of the normal human nasal airway. Br J Pharmacol. 2005; 144(6):867–874

[3] Wise SK, Lin SY, Toskala E, et al. International Consensus Statement on Allergy and Rhinology: Allergic Rhinitis. Int Forum Allergy Rhinol. 2018; 8(2):108–352

23 Corticosteroids

Christine B. Franzese

23.1 Another Major Workhorse

Corticosteroids are highly effective at controlling allergy symptoms and play an integral role in treating allergies. This chapter reviews intranasal, oral, and ocular corticosteroids. It does not cover inhaled or topical corticosteroids.

23.2 What Is This Class of Medication?

These are potent anti-inflammatory medications that result in significant reductions in the release of chemical mediators and decreased recruitment of basophils, eosinophils, and mononuclear cells. These are not histamine blockers and generally do not impact allergy skin testing, with the exception of topical steroids applied to the skin area to be tested.

23.3 What Symptoms Are Good for Treating?

Intranasal corticosteroids: Nasal congestion, rhinorrhea, sneezing, nasal itching, ocular itching, tearing, redness, swelling

Recommended for daily use, there are data that support effectiveness with as needed use.

Oral corticosteroids: Nasal congestion, rhinorrhea, sneezing, nasal and systemic itching, hives, ocular itching, tearing, redness, swelling
Ocular corticosteroids: Tearing, swelling, redness, itching

23.4 Examples of This Class

Intranasal corticosteroids: Fluticasone, flunisolide, mometasone, ciclesonide, budesonide
Oral corticosteroids: Prednisone, methylprednisolone, cortisone, dexamethasone
Ocular corticosteroids: Prednisolone 1%, loteprednol 0.2%, fluorometholone 0.1%

Prednisolone has the greatest anti-inflammatory effect. Fluoromethalone is best for avoiding increased intraocular pressure. Also, consider "soft steroid" eye drops, such as loteprednol. These are new steroid preparations with lower toxicity, better side-effect profile when use is prolonged.

23.5 Why and When to Use

Intranasal corticosteroids: Highly effective at controlling nasal symptoms. When primary complaints focus on nasal congestion, consider using these over oral antihistamines; safe for daily use. If epistaxis develops, inquire if the patient is using correct technique to spray. Avoid in patients with history of severe or chronic epistaxis.

Oral corticosteroids: For allergies, these medications are only used when symptoms are severe and patients are resistant to other medications. These medicines are used only for short period of time because of their side effects and risk profile; not for chronic or daily use.

Ocular corticosteroids: These drops are used for severe eye symptoms, eye symptoms that are resistant or unresponsive to other medications. However, try to avoid chronic long-term use.

23.6 Risks and Side Effects

Intranasal corticosteroids: Nasal dryness and irritation, epistaxis, headache, burning, stinging, septal perforation, possible concerns in pediatric patients regarding reduction in growth velocity.

Take time to educate patients on the proper way to spray nasal steroids. This will help reduce complaints of epistaxis and improve symptom. A good technique is to tell the patient, when spraying into their right nostril, to hold the bottle in their left hand and tilt the nozzle toward the outer corner of their right eye, and vice versa for the left nostril. This gets the medication on the turbinates and avoids deposition on the nasal septum.

Oral corticosteroids: Numerous short-term and long-term risks include hypertension, insomnia, weight gain, hypothalamic-pituitary axis suppression, effects on growth and the musculoskeletal system, hyperglycemia, osteoporosis, aseptic femoral necrosis, anxiety, psychosis, and other side effects.

Ocular corticosteroids: Cataracts, glaucoma/elevated intraocular pressure, risk of viral and fungal infections with prolonged use, corneal-scleral melting

23.7 A Word of Caution About Injectable Corticosteroid Preparations

Injectable steroid preparations have been used to treat symptoms of allergic rhinitis either as intramuscular injections or injections into the inferior turbinate. For intramuscular injections, there is evidence that these provide symptom relief, but have a similar serious side-effect profile to oral steroids without any evidence of increased efficacy. These injections are not recommended unless patients have failed to respond to other treatments and continue to have severe symptoms. While there is evidence that intraturbinate injections are effective in treating symptoms of rhinitis, these types of injections are also accompanied by the rare, but very real, risk of permanent blindness. Other reported side effects include transient blindness, double vision, blurred vision, and medial rectus paralysis. Be sure to carefully weigh the risks and benefits for each of these and that the patient is fully aware of all the risks.

23.8 Age for FDA On-Label Use

Intranasal corticosteroids: Fluticasone (4 years onward), flunisolide (6 years onward), mometasone (2 years onward), ciclesonide (12 years onward), budesonide (6 years onward)

Oral corticosteroids: Age restrictions vary widely depending on reason for use

Ocular corticosteroids: Prednisolone (6 years onward), loteprednol (18 years onward), fluorometholone (2 years onward)

Clinical Pearls	M!

- Good for all allergic symptoms including congestion; use if nasal congestion tends to be a dominant symptom.
- Be sure to advise patients about side effects.
- Be sure to educate patients about the correct spray technique if using intranasal steroid sprays; stop if epistaxis develops.

Bibliography

[1] Bielory L, Katelaris CH, Lightman S, Naclerio RM. Treating the ocular component of allergic rhino-conjunctivitis and related eye disorders. MedGenMed. 2007; 9(3):35

[2] Herman H. Once-daily administration of intranasal corticosteroids for allergic rhinitis: a comparative review of efficacy, safety, patient preference, and cost. Am J Rhinol. 2007; 21(1):70–79

[3] Wise SK, Lin SY, Toskala E, et al. International Consensus Statement on Allergy and Rhinology: Allergic Rhinitis. Int Forum Allergy Rhinol. 2018; 8(2):108–352

24 Leukotriene Receptor Antagonists

Sarah K. Wise

24.1 Most Interesting Information

Leukotrienes mediate many of the unwelcome symptoms of allergy and asthma, such as increased mucus secretion, decreased mucus clearance, and smooth muscle contraction causing bronchoconstriction. Certain drugs have been developed to block leukotriene receptors (i.e., montelukast, zafirlukast) or to inhibit leukotriene synthesis (i.e., zileuton). These drugs have been tested in asthma and allergy, and have shown some benefit. For allergic rhinitis, drugs that block leukotriene receptors are typically not intended as sole therapy. There are certain adverse effects with the leukotriene-modifying agents, so the provider should be educated and be aware before prescribing.

24.2 Serious Stuff

24.2.1 What Are Leukotrienes? (i.e., back to biochemistry class...)

The cys-leukotrienes are produced in leukocytes (especially mast cells and eosinophils), through the arachidonic acid pathway, by the enzyme 5-lipoxygenase. There are various isoforms of cys-leukotrienes, labeled by an alphabet soup (LTA_4, LTC_4, LTD_4, LTE_4). The $cysLT_1$ receptor is found in bronchial mucosa and lung fibroblasts, and has a high affinity for LTD_4. The $cysLT_2$ receptor, where both LTC_4 and LTD_4 act, is found on endothelial cells, leukocytes, lung fibroblasts, and smooth muscle cells. LTB_4 is a bit different, because it is produced from LTA_4 by a hydrolase and acts on receptors BLT_1 and BLT_2. The BLT receptors are found on polymorphonuclear leukocytes and many tissues. The role of LTB_4 and the BLT receptors has been studied less.

24.2.2 Now That the Science Is Over, Why Do We Care About Leukotrienes in Allergy?

Increased mucus secretion, smooth muscle contraction (i.e., bronchoconstriction), and decreased mucociliary clearance are largely initiated by cys-leukotriene release from mast cells in response to allergen. Also, via a positive feedback loop, eosinophils are recruited to target tissues by cys-leukotrienes produced by the eosinophils and mast cells, resulting in increased production of cys-leukotriene. The leukotrienes are, therefore, important mediators of undesirable symptoms in allergy and asthma.

24.2.3 What Are Leukotriene Receptor Antagonists?

Some drugs have been developed that block the $cysLT_1$ receptor, thus reducing the deleterious effects of leukotrienes. These selective $cysLT_1$ receptor antagonists include montelukast and zafirlukast and are taken orally.

In asthma, these drugs demonstrate reduced use of β2-agonist rescue inhalers, reduced nighttime awakenings, some improvement in lung function, decreased health care utilization, and decreased absenteeism. Leukotriene receptor antagonists (LTRAs) are typically recommended as add-on therapy to inhaled corticosteroids in asthma, since the benefit of LTRAs appears to be less than that of inhaled corticosteroids. It is important to remember that all asthma is not the same—the benefit of LTRAs appears to be the best in atopic asthma, pediatric asthma, and exercise-induced bronchospasm.

In allergic rhinitis, level 1 evidence (including at least 13 randomized controlled trials and 6 systematic reviews of randomized controlled trials) demonstrates that LTRAs are superior to placebo for symptom control and improved quality of life (QoL). This effect has been shown in seasonal and perennial allergic rhinitis, as well as in studies-controlled allergen exposure. See later (▶ Section 24.2.6) for comparative effectiveness data versus other available allergic rhinitis medications.

24.2.4 For Completeness Sake… What Is a "Synthesis Inhibitor?"

Zileuton inhibits the 5-lipoxygenase enzyme, thus blocking the production of the cys-leukotrienes. Therefore, zileuton acts much earlier in the arachidonic acid pathway, rather than blocking the leukotriene receptor like LTRAs. Zileuton can suppress allergen-induced eosinophilia and has been shown to improve acute and chronic lung function in asthma. Zileuton can also decrease asthma symptom scores and rescue β2-agonist use. Zileuton is not typically used in the treatment of allergic rhinitis alone.

24.2.5 What Allergic Conditions Can Leukotriene Receptor Antagonists Treat?

Several studies have been conducted on the efficacy of LTRAs for the treatment of allergic rhinitis. In the United States, montelukast is approved by the FDA for the treatment of seasonal and perennial allergic rhinitis in adults. In children with seasonal allergic rhinitis, montelukast is approved down to the age of 2 years. For perennial allergic rhinitis, montelukast is approved down to the age of 6 years.

24.2.6 How Do Leukotriene Receptor Antagonists Compare to Other Allergic Rhinitis Medications?

While LTRAs have shown clear symptom and QoL benefit compared to placebo, current evidence demonstrates that LTRAs are inferior to intranasal corticosteroids for the improvement of symptoms and QoL in the treatment of allergic rhinitis. Compared to oral antihistamines, LTRAs have an equivalent or inferior efficacy for the treatment of allergic rhinitis. When cost is considered, LTRAs are more expensive than many intranasal corticosteroid or oral nonsedating antihistamine preparations. For these reasons, LTRAs are not recommended as first-line single agents for the treatment of allergic rhinitis.

24.2.7 What Is the Best Way to Use Leukotriene Receptor Antagonists?

As stated previously (▶ Section 24.2.6), considering efficacy and cost implications, LTRAs are not recommended as first-choice monotherapy for the treatment of allergic rhinitis. However, in the rare allergic rhinitis patient who cannot take or tolerate intranasal corticosteroids or oral nonsedating antihistamines, LTRAs may be considered as sole therapy. More commonly, LTRAs may be used as add-on therapy in the treatment of allergic rhinitis when first-line medications fail to control symptoms.

Allergic rhinitis and asthma commonly occur together, supporting the unified airway concept. In fact, the 2018 International Consensus Statement for Allergy and Rhinology: Allergic Rhinitis and the 2015 American Academy of Otolaryngology—Head and Neck Surgery Clinical Practice Guideline for Allergic Rhinitis emphasized the importance of assessment of comorbidities in allergic rhinitis. Like allergic rhinitis, however, LTRAs are not recommended over other first-line therapies for asthma. It is better to treat asthma with an inhaled corticosteroid as initial medication, than to choose an LTRA as sole initial therapy. LTRAs may also be considered as add-on therapy for patients with concomitant allergic rhinitis and asthma.

24.2.8 Buyer (and Medical Provider) Beware! What Are the Adverse Effects of Leukotriene Receptor Antagonists?

Like any pharmacotherapy, LTRAs have some adverse effects. These may include:
• Gastrointestinal effects (stomach ache, nausea, diarrhea, heartburn).
• Headache.
• Fatigue or tiredness.

- Tooth pain.
- Sore throat, cough, hoarseness.
- Mood changes, depression (possible increased risk of suicide), anxiety.

There's a black box warning on these medications for neuropsychiatric/behavioral changes. These drugs are very safe, but be sure to inform patients/parent to watch for this side effect.

- Insomnia.
- Skin rash.
- Worsening asthma or trouble breathing (zafirlukast).
- Increased bruising or bleeding, hemoptysis, hematemesis (zafirlukast).
- Impaired liver function (zafirlukast).

Clinical Pearls   M!

- Leukotrienes are responsible for many of the symptoms of allergic rhinitis and asthma.
- Leukotriene receptor antagonists (LTRAs) have demonstrated efficacy in controlling symptoms and improving QoL in allergic rhinitis patients.
- For the treatment of allergic rhinitis, LTRAs are not as efficacious as intra-nasal corticosteroids and have equivalent-to-inferior efficacy compared to oral antihistamines. Considering the cost of these medications and their comparative efficacy, LTRAs are not recommended as first-line single therapy for allergic rhinitis.

Bibliography

[1] Pyasi K, Tufvesson E, Moitra S. Evaluating the role of leukotriene-modifying drugs in asthma management: are their benefits "losing in translation"? Pulm Pharmacol Ther. 2016; 41:52–59

[2] Seidman MD, Gurgel RK, Lin SY, et al. Guideline Otolaryngology Development Group. AAO-HNSF. Clinical practice guideline: allergic rhinitis. Otolaryngol Head Neck Surg. 2015; 152(1) Suppl:S1–S43

[3] Wise SK, Lin SY, Toskala E, et al. International Consensus Statement on Allergy and Rhinology: Allergic Rhinitis. Int Forum Allergy Rhinol. 2018; 8(2):108–352

25 Mast Cell Stabilizers

Sarah K. Wise

25.1 Preventing Degranulation

During ancient times cromolyn-like products were used. Nowadays various mast cell stabilizing products are available to treat allergic conditions. Their primary mechanism of action is thought to be mast cell stabilization, or inhibition of mast cell degranulation, although additional benefits are likely derived from effects on other cellular mediators in the allergic cascade. Cromolyn and cromolyn-like products are safe, efficacious, and generally well tolerated; however, their short half-life requires frequent dosing.

25.2 Serious Stuff

25.2.1 What Is Cromolyn?

Cromolyn and cromolyn-like products, such as disodium cromoglycate (DSCG), are inspired by the mast cell-stabilizing properties of Khellin, derived from a plant called *Ammi visnaga*. It is spasmolytic and its use dates back to ancient Egyptian times. You may see various names for cromolyn-type products such as DSCG, cromolyn sodium, sodium cromoglycate, disodium 4,4′-dioxo-5, 5′-(2-hydroxytrimethylenedioxy)-di(4H-chromene-2-carboxylate).

Although the mechanism of cromolyn's effect is somewhat debated, it is thought to stabilize mast cells by altering the function of cellular chloride channels. This prevents influx of calcium into the cytoplasm from the extracellular space, and ultimately stops degranulation of the sensitized mast cell, which would typically occur following cross-linking of mast cell-bound allergen-specific immunoglobulin E (IgE) that has come into contact with its antigen. If the mast cell does not degranulate, histamine is not released. In addition, if calcium influx is stopped, synthesis of lipid mediators such as prostaglandins and leukotrienes is affected, along with other cytokines and chemokines.

First-generation mast cell stabilizers DSCG and nedocromil sodium prevent mast cell degranulation. Later generation mast cell-stabilizing products such as olopatadine also contain antihistamines, giving them an added benefit in the treatment of allergic disease. Various cromolyn-like products also have apparent effects on eosinophils, macrophages, monocytes, that increase their anti-allergy properties. Chromolyn-type products work on both the early- and late-phase allergic responses.

25.2.2 What Allergic Conditions Can Mast Cell Stabilizers Treat?

Mast cell stabilizing-products are available as topical or inhaled preparations for allergic rhinitis and asthma. Combination mast cell stabilizer and antihistamine products are a first-line therapy for seasonal and perennial allergic conjunctivitis, as well as maintenance treatment for vernal keratoconjunctivitis and atopic keratoconjunctivitis. Oral formulations may also be used to control certain allergic food reactions.

- **Some cromolyn-type products:** DSCG, cromolyn sodium, nedocromil sodium, lodoxamide tromethamine, olopatadine, pemirolast

25.2.3 What Is the Best Way to Use Cromolyn Products?

Since cromolyn's primary mechanism of action is thought to be inhibition of mast cell degranulation, typical recommendations are for the use of these products before the onset of allergic symptoms. In other words, while cromolyn-type products may be used at various times in the allergic disease process, prophylactic use is the best way to succeed with these medications.

25.2.4 What's So Great About Mast Cell Stabilizers?

Cromolyn-type products are safe and some preparations may be used in very young patients (down to the age of 2 years; check specific product labeling and indications). These medications work especially well for seasonal allergic rhinitis. DSCG has been shown to decrease nasal congestion, rhinorrhea, and sneezing. There is efficacy demonstrated over placebo.

25.2.5 What Is *Not* So Great About Mast Cell Stabilizers?

DSCG has a short half-life. It requires frequent dosing, which may affect compliance. Nasal or nasopharyngeal irritation, epistaxis, foul taste, and sneezing are some of adverse effects. Studies conducted on the use of cromolyn-type products in perennial allergic rhinitis are less convincing of benefit, compared to seasonal allergic rhinitis. It is also clear that for allergic rhinitis, cromolyn-type products do not work as well as intranasal corticosteroids. Currently, there are no studies that compare cromolyn to intranasal antihistamines in the allergic rhinitis population.

Clinical Pearls M!

- Cromolyn products are thought to have a primary mechanism of inhibition of mast cell degranulation, although some other cellular mechanisms likely contribute as well.
- In seasonal allergic rhinitis, DSCG has demonstrated efficacy over placebo. However, it has inferior efficacy to intranasal corticosteroids and has not been studied against intranasal antihistamines.
- Cromolyn products are generally safe.
- Certain side effects and the need for frequent dosing may affect compliance with cromolyn products.
- The use of DSCG for allergic rhinitis is considered an option, with the best method being prophylactic use prior to encountering a known allergic trigger.

Bibliography

[1] Ackerman S, Smith LM, Gomes PJ. Ocular itch associated with allergic conjunctivitis: latest evidence and clinical management. Ther Adv Chronic Dis. 2016; 7(1):52–67

[2] Finn DF, Walsh JJ. Twenty-first century mast cell stabilizers. Br J Pharmacol. 2013; 170(1):23–37

[3] Mantelli F, Calder VL, Bonini S. The anti-inflammatory effects of therapies for ocular allergy. J Ocul Pharmacol Ther. 2013; 29(9):786–793

[4] Ridolo E, Montagni M, Melli V, Braido F, Incorvaia C, Canonica GW. Pharmacotherapy of allergic rhinitis: current options and future perspectives. Expert Opin Pharmacother. 2014; 15(1):73–83

[5] Wise SK, Lin SY, Toskala E, et al. International Consensus Statement on Allergy and Rhinology: Allergic Rhinitis. Int Forum Allergy Rhinol. 2018; 8(2):108–352

26 Combination Therapies

Sarah K. Wise

26.1 Working Together

Various pharmacotherapy combinations are used clinically to control allergic rhinitis symptoms. Many of these combinations have been evaluated in randomized controlled trials and systematic reviews. Interestingly, some of the most common medication combinations used to treat allergic rhinitis symptoms do not have strong supporting evidence.

26.2 Serious Stuff

26.2.1 What Are Combination Therapies?

Ideally, when treating any medical condition, appropriate relief would be obtained with a single intervention. However, this may not always be the case. Combination therapies are frequently used to treat allergic rhinitis for various reasons. Perhaps a single medication does not adequately control symptoms, and the addition of a second medication provides further symptom reduction. Or, one medication may work well for certain allergic rhinitis symptoms, and a different medication may aid in reducing other symptoms. Whatever the case, several medications may be used in combination to treat allergic rhinitis. This chapter considers some of the most common medication combinations for allergic rhinitis, along with the benefits and downsides of each combination.

26.2.2 Lay It out for Me. Give Me the High Points. Just the Facts, Ma'am. What Do I Really Need to Know?

▶ Table 26.1 succinctly reviews four of the most common medication combinations used to treat allergic rhinitis. This is meant to be a quick review of issues to consider when choosing a medication combination.

Table 26.1 Four common medication combinations and their pros/cons

Medication 1 (examples)	Medication 2 (examples)	Benefits	Downsides	Succinct recommendations
Oral antihistamine (cetirizine, loratadine, fexofenadine)	Oral decongestant (pseudoephedrine)	Unrelated mechanism of two drugs provides synergy. Controls sneezing, itching, and nasal congestion. Improved control of nasal congestion vs. antihistamine alone. Combination is more effective for reducing symptoms in SAR than either drug alone.	Oral decongestant side effects: Systemic hypertension, urinary retention (additional adverse effects noted in pregnant women and young children). Drug-drug interactions for oral antihistamines are prevalent, especially in elderly.	Typically considered an option for acute AR exacerbations, but not recommended as daily maintenance therapy.
Oral antihistamine (cetirizine, loratadine, fexofenadine)	Oral LTRA (montelukast)	Oral antihistamine plus LTRA improves symptoms and QoL compared to placebo.	Current evidence is variable regarding combination oral antihistamine and LTRA versus either drug alone. Current evidence indicates that combination oral antihistamine and LTRA is inferior to INCS for AR symptom control.	An effective INCS appears to be a better choice for AR symptom control, compared to combination oral antihistamine and LTRA. If a patient cannot tolerate INCS, or has comorbid asthma, this combination is an option.

(Continued) ▶

Table 26.1 (continued)

Medication 1 (examples)	Medication 2 (examples)	Benefits	Downsides	Succinct recommendations
Oral antihistamine (cetirizine, loratadine, fexofenadine)	INCS (fluticasone propionate, mometasone furoate)	Addition of INCS when a patient is already taking an oral antihistamine provides symptom improvement, especially for nasal congestion.	Most studies show no benefit of adding an oral antihistamine to INCS, compared to an effective INCS alone.	Although this combination is often used clinically, based on current evidence, if a patient is already on an effective INCS, adding an oral antihistamine provides no additional benefit. The key medication in this combination is an effective INCS.
Intranasal antihistamine (azelastine, olopatadine)	INCS (fluticasone propionate, mometasone furoate)	Quick onset of action. Improved symptom control for AR vs. either medication alone.	Foul taste due to intranasal antihistamine component. Increased financial burden.	When considering an addition of an antihistamine to INCS, evidence supports an intranasal antihistamine over an oral antihistamine. This combination is typically considered second-line therapy when symptoms not controlled by either medication alone.

Abbreviations: AR, allergic rhinitis; INCS, intranasal corticosteroid; LTRA, leukotriene receptor antagonist; QoL, quality of life; SAR, seasonal allergic rhinitis.

Clinical Pearls   **M!**

- Various combinations of medications are used to treat allergic rhinitis.
- An oral antihistamine and oral decongestant combination provides synergistic symptom benefit in allergic rhinitis and is generally recommended for acute symptom exacerbations.
- An INCS and intranasal antihistamine combination is beneficial. When considering an addition of an antihistamine to an INCS, the patient will likely benefit more from adding an intranasal antihistamine rather than an oral antihistamine.

Bibliography

[1] Wise SK, Lin SY, Toskala E, et al. International Consensus Statement on Allergy and Rhinology: Allergic Rhinitis. Int Forum Allergy Rhinol. 2018; 8(2):108–352

27 Biologics

Cecelia C. Damask

27.1 Introduction to Biologics

Allergic disorders including atopic dermatitis (AD) and asthma have a high prevalence, but even with prevailing available therapies, many patients continue to have uncontrolled symptoms. Although some patients present with similar clinical symptoms, the drivers of their disease processes can be different. This has brought the concept of endotyping to the forefront of our understanding of these diseases. An endotype is a subclassification of a particular disease that is based on a particular pathophysiologic mechanism and associated clinical biomarkers. Targeted therapies are available based on specific endotypes. There are two inflammatory pathways that drive allergic disease: Type 2 (T_h2) inflammation and non-type 2 inflammation. All of the biologics currently approved for use focus on the T_h-2 inflammatory pathway. Targets along this pathway include anti-interleukin (IL)-5, anti-immunoglobulin E (IgE), anti-IL-4, and anti-IL-13. This chapter also reviews the current use of biologics in allergic disorders. See ► Table 27.1 for a summary of trials using monoclonal antibodies.

27.2 Immunoglobulin E

27.2.1 Omalizumab

Omalizumab targets circulating IgE. In 2003, omalizumab became the first Food and Drug Administration (FDA)-approved biologic for use in moderate to severe asthma. Mast cells and basophils have high-affinity IgE receptors (FcεR1) on them. Omalizumab is a recombinant humanized anti-IgE antibody that blocks IgE from binding to these high-affinity receptors, thus blunting the allergic response that would be driven by the release of histamines, prostaglandins, leukotrienes, and other mediators.

Omalizumab was first approved for use in adults and adolescents (12 years of age and above) with moderate to severe persistent asthma. The large trials showed that omalizumab reduced asthma exacerbations. Patients in the studies had a serum IgE level between 30 and 700 IU/mL and a positive skin test or in vitro reactivity to a perennial aeroallergen. In 2016, it became approved for children aged between 6 and 12 years for uncontrolled moderate- to severe-persistent allergic asthma.

In 2014, the FDA-approved omalizumab for the indication of chronic idiopathic urticaria (CIU) in patients aged 12 years and up who remain symptomatic despite treatment with antihistamines.

Table 27.1

Monoclonal Antibody	Mechanism of Action	Indication	Patient Type	Status	Dosing
Asthma					
Omalizumab	IgE (at Fcε3)	Moderate to severe persistent asthma in patients 6 years of age and older with a positive skin test or in vitro reactivity to a perennial aeroallergen and symptoms that are inadequately controlled with inhaled corticosteroids	IgE 30-700, + SPT or in vitro for at least one perennial aeroallergen	Approved	SC q 2-4 weeks based on IgE and weight
Mepolizumab	IL-5	Severe asthma aged 12 years and older with an eosinophilic phenotype	Blood eos > 300 within 12 months of enrollment Blood eosinophil level ≥ 150 at initiation of treatment (w/in 6 months of dosing)	Approved	SC q 4 weeks
Reslizumab	IL-5	Severe asthma aged 18 years and older with an eosinophilic phenotype	Septum eos > 3%	Approved	IV q 4 weeks
Benralizumab	IL-5Rα	Severe asthma aged 12 years and older with an eosinophilic phenotype	Severe asthma, > 1 exacerbation a year Eos > 300	Approved	SC q 8 weeks (first 3 doses monthly)

(Continued) ▶

Table 27.1 (continued)

Monoclonal Antibody	Mechanism of Action	Indication	Patient Type	Status	Dosing
Dupilumab	IL-4Rα	Moderate-to-severe asthma aged 12 years and older with an eosinophilic phenotype or with oral corticosteroid dependent asthma	Moderate to severe asthma with an eosinophilic phenotype or PO corticosteroid dependent asthma (eos > 150 of FeNO > 25)	Phase 3 completed	SC q 2 weeks
Lebrikizumab	IL-13		Severe asthma, > 1 exacerbation a year	Phase 3 completed	
Tralokinumab	IL-13		Severe asthma; recurrent exacerbations	Phase 3 underway	
Tezepelumab	TSLP		Mild allergic asthma	Phase 3 underway	
Navarixin	CXCR2 Receptor Antagonist		Sputum neutrophils > 40%	Phase 2 completed	
Atopic Dermatitis					
Dupilumab	IL-4Rα	Moderate-to-severe atopic dermatitis aged 12 years and older whose disease is not adequately controlled with topical prescription therapies or when those therapies are not advisable	Moderate to severe Atopic Dermatitis	Approved	SC q 2 weeks
Lebrikizumab	IL-13		Moderate to severe Atopic Dermatitis	Phase 2 underway	

Table 27.1 (continued)

Monoclonal Antibody	Mechanism of Action	Indication	Patient Type	Status	Dosing
Tralokinumab	IL-13		Moderate to severe Atopic Dermatitis	Phase 3 underway	
Omalizumab	IgE		Moderate to severe Atopic Dermatitis	Phase 2 completed	
Mepolizumab	IL-5		Atopic Dermatitis	Phase 2 completed	
Nemolizumab	IL-31		Atopic Dermatitis	Phase 2 completed	
Chronic Idiopathic Urticaria (CIU)					
Omalizumab	IgE	Patients aged 12 years and older who remain symptomatic despite H1 antihistamine treatment	Moderate to severe CIU	Approved	SC q 4 weeks
Eosinophilic Granulomatosis with Polyangitis (EGPA)					
Mepolizumab	IL-5	Adult patients with eosinophilic granulomatosis with polyangitis (EGPA)	EGPA on stable oral steroids	Approved	SC q 4 weeks
Reslizumab	IL-5		EGPA	Phase 2 underway	
Benralizumab	IL-5Rα		EGPA	Phase 2 underway	

(Continued) ▶

Table 27.1 (continued)

Monoclonal Antibody	Mechanism of Action	Indication	Patient Type	Status	Dosing
Eosinolphilic Esophagitis (EoE)					
Mepolizumab	IL-5		Adults with EoE; >20 eos per HPF	Phase 2 underway	
Reslizumab	IL-5		Children & adolescents with EoE; >24 eos per HPF	Phase 2 completed	
Chronic Rhinosinusitis with Nasal Polyps (CRSwNP)					
Omalizumab	IgE		CRSwNP with asthma; IgE 30-700	Phase 3 underway	
Mepolizumab	IL-5		severe CRSwNP	Phase 3 underway	
Reslizumab	IL-5		Massive nasal polyps	Phase 1 completed	
Benralizumab	IL-5Rα		Severe nasal polyposis	Phase 3 underway	
Dupilumab	IL-4Rα		CRSwNP	Phase 3 completed	

Omalizumab was found to improve nasal symptoms in patients with chronic rhinosinusitis with nasal polyposis (CRSwNP). However, this was only studied in CRSwNP patients who also had comorbid asthma. Phase III studies are currently underway investigating use in CRSwNP subjects.

27.2.2 Interleukin-5

Interleukin-5 is a cytokine that is predominately secreted by T lymphocytes, eosinophils, mast cells, and type 2 innate lymphoid cells. Interleukin-5 promotes maturation of eosinophils in the bone marrow, survival and activation of eosinophils as well as cellular differentiation. Interleukin-5 also plays a role in B-cell survival and thus can promote IgE production and subsequent mast cell and basophil activation. Due to the multiple roles of IL-5, it is thought to play a role in hypereosinophilic intrinsic asthma as well as extrinsic allergic asthma. By blocking IL-5, monoclonal antibodies have dramatically changed the management of severe eosinophilic asthma. There are currently three biologics targeting IL-5 activity: Mepolizumab, reslizumab, and benralizumab.

27.2.3 Mepolizumab

Mepolizumab is a humanized monoclonal anti-IL-5 antibody. It has been approved by the FDA in 2015 for use in severe persistent asthmatics aged 12 years and up via subcutaneous injection administered monthly.

In a proof-of-concept study, mepolizumab showed improvement in nasal polyp scores in patients with CRSwNP. At the time of press, a phase III clinical trial for mepolizumab in CRSwNP is underway.

In 2017, the FDA approved mepolizumab for the indication of eosinophilic granulomatosis with polyangiitis (EGPA).

27.2.4 Reslizumab

Reslizumab is a humanized monoclonal antibody directed against IL-5. It is dosed in a weight-based fashion and is administered by intravenous (IV) infusion every 4 weeks at a dose of 3.0 mg/kg. It has been approved by the FDA in 2016 for use in severe eosinophilic asthma in patients aged 18 years and older.

In a proof-of-concept study, reslizumab showed improvement in nasal polyp scores in patients with CRSwNP. At the time of press, no phase III clinical trials for using reslizumab in treating CRSwNP are underway.

27.2.5 Benralizumab

Benralizumab targets IL-5Rα that is found on the surface of eosinophils and basophils. Once it binds to the receptor, it induces apoptosis of that bound cell through activity of natural killer cells. Benralizumab has been approved by the

FDA in 2017 for use in severe persistent eosinophilic asthma in patients aged 12 years and up. After monthly dosing for the first 3 months, benralizumab is administered subcutaneously every 8 weeks.

At the time of press, a phase III clinical trial for benralizumab in CRSwNP is underway.

27.2.6 Interleukin-4 and Interleukin-13

Interleukin-4 plays a role in CD4+ lymphocyte differentiation as well as the production of IgE. Interleukin-13 drives mucus production, airway hyperresponsiveness, and subepithelial fibrosis. Both (IL-4 and IL-13) share a receptor complex (IL-4Rα/IL-13Rα1).

27.2.7 Dupilumab

Dupilumab is a fully humanized monoclonal antibody that binds to the α-subunit of the IL-4 receptor and inhibits both IL-4 and IL-13 activity. Dupilumab has been approved by the FDA in 2017 for use in moderate-to-severe AD when symptoms are inadequately controlled with topical treatments. In 2018, dupilumab was also approved for moderate-to-severe asthma with an eosinophilic phenotype or oral corticosteroid dependency.

Two phase III clinical studies were completed in 2018 evaluating the efficacy of dupilumab in reducing the severity of nasal congestion/obstruction and endoscopic nasal polyp score in adult patients with CRSwNP.

Dupilumab was investigated for use in the treatment of eosinophilic esophagitis (EoE). A phase II study was completed assessing the efficacy in the patients as well as safety. This study revealed improvement in dysphagia scores and peak eosinophil counts.

27.2.8 Librikizumab and Tralokinumab

Both lebrikizumab and tralokinumab are IL-13 antibodies. They are both studied for use in severe persistent asthma. Only one of lebrikizumab's phase III trials met its primary outcomes and both the trials had a high number of adverse events. A statement was released in 2017 that both phase III trials for tralokinumab did not meet their primary endpoints.

27.2.9 Thymic Stromal Lymphopoietin

Thymic stromal lymphopoietin (TSLP) is an epithelial-cell-derived cytokine that drives allergic inflammatory responses through the innate immune system. It activates mast cells and dendritic cells. There is interest in TSLP as a target for asthma treatment.

27.2.10 Tezepelumab

Tezepelumab is a humanized monoclonal antibody that binds to TSLP and prevents interaction with its receptor. A phase II study has been completed that revealed lower rates of asthma exacerbations.

27.3 Interleukin-31

27.3.1 Nemolizumab

Nemolizumab is a humanized antibody against IL-31 receptor A. Interleukin-31 may play a role in the pathobiologic mechanism of AD and more specifically, in the occurrence of pruritus. The IL-31 inhibitor, nemolizumab, significantly improved pruritus in patients with moderate to severe AD in a phase II, randomized, double-blind, placebo-controlled trial. At the time of the writing of this chapter, a phase III study is not yet underway.

27.3.2 What Do We Still Not Know?

1. In patients with type-2 high asthma, what is the best biomarker to predict optimal response to a specific biologic?
2. What is the best way to diagnose and optimally treat type-2 low asthma?

Clinical Pearls   M!

- IgE plays an important role in urticaria and asthma as well as a role in some patients with CRSwNP, thus providing the rationale for the use of omalizumab.
- Blocking IL-5 is an effective treatment in some patients with asthma and CRSwNP.
- Blocking both IL-4 and IL-13 is effective in treating multiple allergic and respiratory diseases, including AD, asthma, and CRSwNP.
- Choosing a biologic for asthma, AD, urticaria, or nasal polyps should be based on disease phenotype, relevant biomarkers, comorbid conditions, and FDA approval status.
- Type-2 high asthma has the most choices of available FDA-approved biologic therapies, including omalizumab, mepolizumab, reslizumab, dupilumab, and benralizumab.
- Omalizumab is the only FDA-approved biologic for chronic idiopathic (spontaneous) urticaria.
- Dupilumab is the only FDA-approved biologic for AD.
- At the time of writing this chapter, no biologics are FDA-approved for CRSwNP. Dupilumab has completed phase III trials and omalizumab, mepolizumab, and benralizumab are undergoing phase III trials.

These atopic disorders pose challenges for physicians. Biologic therapies constitute a truly innovative therapeutic option. With the introduction of these new treatment modalities, it is an exciting time for the physicians to care for their most challenging patients in the field of allergy and asthma.

Bibliography

[1] Bleecker ER, FitzGerald JM, Chanez P, et al. SIROCCO study investigators. Efficacy and safety of benralizumab for patients with severe asthma uncontrolled with high-dosage inhaled corticosteroids and long-acting β2-agonists (SIROCCO): a randomised, multicentre, placebo-controlled phase 3 trial. Lancet. 2016; 388(10056):2115–2127

[2] Casale TB. Biologics and biomarkers for asthma, urticaria, and nasal polyposis. J Allergy Clin Immunol. 2017; 1; 39(5):1411–1421

[3] Hanania NA, Alpan O, Hamilos DL, et al. Omalizumab in severe allergic asthma inadequately controlled with standard therapy: a randomized trial. Ann Intern Med. 2011; 154(9):573–582

[4] Kaplan A, Ledford D, Ashby M, et al. Omalizumab in patients with symptomatic chronic idiopathic/spontaneous urticaria despite standard combination therapy. J Allergy Clin Immunol. 2013; 132(1):101–109

[5] Ortega HG, Liu MC, Pavord ID, et al. MENSA Investigators. Mepolizumab treatment in patients with severe eosinophilic asthma. N Engl J Med. 2014; 371(13):1198–1207

[6] Simpson EL, Bieber T, Guttman-Yassky E, et al. SOLO 1 and SOLO 2 Investigators. Two phase 3 trials of dupilumab versus placebo in atopic dermatitis. N Engl J Med. 2016; 375(24):2335–2348

28 Alternative Remedies

Christine B. Franzese

28.1 The Mind Is a Powerful Thing

The physician should have some out-of-the box knowledge regardless of his/her opinion on alternative remedies. The goal of every physician is to help patients. To provide the best care, a physician should try to balance the knowledge acquired through study, the experience gained through clinical practice, and the evidence that has been evaluated in the literature to make the best possible treatment recommendations. There are still quite a few areas of clinical practice where physicians recommend or prescribe things that are off-label or don't have a lot of thorough evidence behind them. There is also the desire among some patients to avoid pharmaceuticals, to try alternative remedies, or to use "natural" therapies. On one hand, this is very frustrating for a physician, especially when there are treatments to offer backed up by thorough medical evidence; on the other hand, the physician sometimes prescribe off-label treatments they "know" work, but don't have solid proof supporting them.

The author struggles to keep this equilibrium in mind when approaching the patient who is resistant to using traditional therapy. However, being familiar with them can help discuss them with patients and gain their trust. If patients trust the physician, they may listen and the practitioner may have a shot at helping them, rather than letting them walk out of the door thinking they have visited just another "drug pusher."

28.2 Honey/Local Honey/Raw Honey

Honey is the most attractive of all the alternative remedies, not just because it is heard the most, but because of its potential similarity to sublingual allergy treatments. The thought is that locally produced pollens are incorporated into honey and by consuming it regularly an oral tolerance to these allergens develops. However, the types of pollen that tend to cause allergic immunoglobulin E (IgE) sensitization tend to be airborne (anemophilous). The type of pollen collected by insects is entomophilous (insect-borne) pollen which is sticky, heavy, and not thought to cause IgE-mediated respiratory disease.

Honey has been shown to have some antibacterial, wound healing, and general anti-inflammatory effects. The evidence regarding the use of honey to treat allergic rhinitis is equivocal, demonstrating no clear benefit in humans. Reportedly, honey must be consumed daily at high doses to demonstrate health benefits. For European bee honey, the dose should be around 7 teaspoons (50 gm) to 11.5 teaspoons (80 gm).

135

28.3 Risks/Side Effects

- Honey is generally considered safe.
- Be cautious in diabetics/prediabetics due to increases in blood sugar.
- Do not give to children under the age of 1 year because of risks of infantile botulism.
- Mad Honey disease is a risk to humans and animals when consuming unprocessed honey from small batches due to grayanotoxins produced by rhododendrons, azaleas, and some other flowers. Symptoms of Mad Honey disease include dizziness, excessive sweating, nausea, vomiting, hypotension, palpitations, seizures, and rarely death.

28.4 Acupuncture

One of the oldest practiced healing arts, this traditional Chinese medicine focuses on the manipulation of the flows of Qi, the body's vital energy, which travels through a series of lines, or meridians, under the skin. Disease occurs when the flow of Qi is disrupted and by stimulating acupuncture points with needles, disease can be treated by restoring the balance of Qi.

Acupuncture has been shown to have positive effects on other disease process, but has demonstrated no clear benefit for allergic symptoms. While the effects of acupuncture on allergic symptoms have been studied, most of the studies allowed unrestricted use of traditional allergy medications, which makes the evidence difficult to interpret.

28.5 Risks/Side Effects

- Acupuncture is generally considered safe.
- Risks associated with acupuncture are those of needle sticks: Pain, redness, swelling, and infection.

28.6 Herbal Therapies

There are an extensive number of single and combination herbal remedies purported to treat allergies and allergic symptoms. ▶ Table 28.1 is a small list of just a few of the most common ones. Some of these have been evaluated in studies, but the studies are either small, of poor quality, with contradictory findings, or have findings that have not been replicated. Although there has been no conclusive evidence to support the recommendation of any of these, there is one in particular that has been mentioned in this chapter, because the author occasionally recommends it to some allergy patients who also have migraines.

Table 28.1 List of herbal remedies reported to be used to treat allergy symptoms

Butterbur (*Petasites hybridus*), Capsaicin
Huang qi (*Astragalus membranaceus*), Benifuuki green tea
Grape seed extract, Beefsteak plant (*Perilla frutescens*)
Ten-Cha (*Rubus suavissimus*), Tinofend (*Tinospora cordifolia*)
Stinging nettle (*Urtica dioica*), Indian gooseberry (*Phyllanthus emblica*)
Myrobalan (*Terminalia chebula*), Bahera (*Terminalia chebula*)
East Indian walnut tree (*Albizia labbeck*), Ginger (*Zingiber officinale*)
Long pepper (*Piper longum*), Black pepper (*Piper nigrum*)
Ginkgo (*Ginkgo biloba*), Chinese skullcap (*Scutellaria baicalensis*)
Horny goat weed (*Epimedium sagittatum*), Japanese apricot (*Prunus mume*)

Butterbur seems to have antihistaminic, antileukotriene, and mast cell inhibitory effects. It is also recommended as a potential complementary treatment option in guidelines for adult episodic migraines released by the American Academy of Neurology and the American Headache Society. There is some evidence supporting its effectiveness in treating allergy symptoms, but not enough to demonstrate it as clearly beneficial or superior. However, in patients with migraines who are potentially interested in complementary therapy, this option may help them in treating their migraines and allergies.

28.7 Risks/Side Effects

- Parts of the butterbur plant contain pyrrolizidine alkaloids (PAs). These are toxic compounds that cause liver, lung, and cardiovascular damage, as well as potentially be carcinogenic. Preparations must come from a reputable supplier and be certified "PA Free."
- Use with caution and per instructions on the bottle.
- Use no more than 16 weeks—safety beyond this is unclear.

Clinical Pearls	M!
- Even if a practitioner doesn't recommend any of the above, he/she should be familiar with them. This will help further conversations with patients and offers some chance to educate them.	

Bibliography

[1] Chawla J. Migraine Headache Guidelines. Available at https://emedicine.medscape.com/article/1142556-guidelines. Accessed July 1, 2018

[2] Jansen SA, Kleerekooper I, Hofman ZLM, Kappen IF, Stary-Weinzinger A, van der Heyden MA. Grayanotoxin poisoning: 'mad honey disease' and beyond. Cardiovasc Toxicol. 2012; 12(3):208–215

[3] Wise SK, Lin SY, Toskala E, et al. International Consensus Statement on Allergy and Rhinology: Allergic Rhinitis. Int Forum Allergy Rhinol. 2018; 8(2):108–352

29 Immunotherapy: Subcutaneous Immunotherapy

Cecelia C. Damask, Christine B. Franzese

29.1 The Basics of Subcutaneous Immunotherapy

Once the decision is made to treat and the relevant positive allergy tests (in vitro and/or skin tests) are evaluated and correlated with the patient's symptomatology, one or more treatment vials are created according to a prescription or "recipe" the provider creates (see Chapter 45 on candidate selection for further discussion on selecting candidates for subcutaneous immunotherapy [SCIT]). During escalation and maintenance, usually 5 mL multiallergen, mutidose vials are mixed, each of which contains 10 doses of 0.50 mL volume.

> If 10 mL vials are used, then there's generally 10 doses of 1.0 mL volume. This chapter will focus on 5-mL vial creation.

29.2 To Endpoint or Not to Endpoint

A vial prescription or "recipe" can be created using an "endpoint" to determine a starting dilution for treatment. See Chapter 16 on the definition of an endpoint and how it's determined. If using an endpoint, the initial treatment vial begins at a treatment dose for each antigen equal to 0.05 mL of the endpoint dilution and escalates to a maximum dose of 0.50 mL.

> If you are not using an endpoint to determine a starting point for treatment, then generally the weakest dilution prepared is used. In some practices, all antigens may start at a #6 dilution, in other practices it may be a #4 dilution. If you are just beginning to add allergy to your practice, using the weakest dilution (#6) is recommended until more experience is gained.

Volume reduction is accomplished by using dilutions that are 25 times more concentrated than the endpoint, commonly referred to as "two dilutions to the right." To prepare 10 doses would require 10 × 0.50 mL, or 5 mL of the endpoint dilution for the maximum dose for each antigen. This is equal to 1 mL of the next more concentrated dilution, or 0.20 mL of the solution that is two dilutions more concentrated. Therefore, a treatment vial for a patient is created by adding 0.20 mL for each antigen, taken for a dilution that is 25 times more concentrated than the endpoint dilution, and the total volume is adjusted to equal 5 mL by adding appropriate amounts of glycerin and phenolated normal saline (PNS) diluent.

29.3 Can You Say That Again?

If the endpoint for cat was #6 and the practitioner adds cat to the treatment vial, he/she should add 0.20 mL of #4 cat to the vial. Add 0.20 mL two dilutions "to the right" (stronger) of each additional allergen that you want in the vial then add enough diluent to bring the volume up to 5 mL (▶ Table 29.1).

29.4 A Few Words About Preservatives

There are several factors that can influence the loss of potency over time. Storage temperature is important. Patient vials and practitioner's "concentrates" should be stored between 2 and 8 °C. Stabilizers and bactericidal agents can also influence potency. There are several additives that can be used in patient vials; these include phenol, human serum albumin (HSA), and glycerin. There are few studies on potency. Therefore, recommendations regarding which preservative to use and expiration dates are not strongly evidence-based.

If PNS is used as a diluent, the potency of the extracts in that vial will last about 6 to 8 weeks even if refrigerated. However, if a 10% glycerin concentration is added, the potency will last about 12 weeks. A 10% glycerin concentration in a patient vial can be achieved by adding 1 mL of 50% glycerin to the vial.

Table 29.1 Example of simple SCIT vial prescription

Antigen	Endpoint	Volume	"Two dilutions to the right"
Cat	#6	0.20 mL	#4
Dog	#4	0.20 mL	#2
Oak	#2	0.20 mL	Conc
Ragweed	#6	0.20 mL	#4
Add diluent		4.2 mL	
To make total		5.0 mL	

1 mL of 50% glycerin added to 4 mL of PNS equals 10% glycerin concentration achieved in the vial.

Human serum albumin also makes a great preservative choice. Some studies have shown evidence that it is a superior allergen extract stabilizer, especially with very dilute extracts. It also inhibits protein aggregation.

29.5 Recipe Examples

Refer to ▶ Table 29.2 for dilution preparations.

29.6 Serious Stuff: Vial Mixing

Any type of allergy vial mixing, whether it is for preparation of a testing/treatment board or for patient vials for sublingual immunotherapy (SLIT) or SCIT therapy or even for oral mucosal immunotherapy (OMIT) toothpaste preparation, falls under United States Pharmacopeia (USP) 797 guidelines that contain the standards for preparing compounded sterile drugs. Please see Chapter 43 for further discussion on these requirements for space, sterility measures, compounding staff training and responsibilities, and environmental monitoring.

29.7 Tools of the Trade (What All Are Needed)

- Antigens ("concentrates") from the manufacturer.
- Sterile empty 5 mL vials to be used when preparing the individual patient vials.
- 23 gauge needles.
- Diluent.
  - The practitioner may choose to use PNS.
  - The practitioner may choose to use HSA.
- 50% glycerin (unless HSA is being used as diluent/preservative).
- Labels for the patient vials.

Table 29.2 Examples of SCIT vial prescriptions using different diluents

Using PNS as diluent with 1 mL of 50% glycerin			
Antigen	Endpoint	Volume	"Two dilutions to the right"
Cat	#6	0.20 mL	#4
Dog	#4	0.20 mL	#2
Oak	#2	0.20 mL	Conc
Ragweed	#6	0.20 mL	#4
Add 50% glycerin		1.0 mL	
Add diluent		3.2 mL	
To make total		5.0 mL	

Using HSA as diluent			
Antigen	Endpoint	Volume	"Two dilutions to the right"
Cat	#6	0.20 mL	#4
Dog	#4	0.20 mL	#2
Oak	#2	0.20 mL	Conc
Ragweed	#6	0.20 mL	#4
Add HSA diluent		4.2 mL	
To make total		5.0 mL	

Abbreviations: HSA, human serum albumin; PNS, phenolated normal saline.

29.8 Shocking Information (How to Actually Do This!)

Step 1: Create the SCIT prescription.
- Correlate the patient's symptoms to their testing results and decide which antigens are to be treated.
- On a mixing form/SCIT prescription form, write the order to add each antigen you want to include at 0.2 mL two dilutions "to the right" (stronger).
- Add up the volume of all the antigens that need to be treated in one vial.
- Calculate in 1 mL of 50% glycerin.

> Antigen concentrate contains 50% glycerin, so 0.2 mL of antigen concentrate is equal to 0.2 mL of 50% glycerin as well. Be sure to factor this into your calculations. If using 5 or more concentrates in a vial, you've already added 1 mL of glycerin, so no additional glycerin is needed.
>
> HSA is a great preservative. If HSA is being used as a diluent, do not need to add any additional glycerin.

- Then calculate the remaining volume that would be needed to bring the total up to 5 mL and add in this amount of diluent (either PNS or HSA).

Step 2: Label the vials.
- Print labels and affix them to the sterile empty patient vials.
- Make sure to have two patient identifiers on the vial (name and date of birth).
- Also include the use by date (UBD) on the vials.
- Include storage instructions such as "store between 2 and 8 °C."

Step 3: Follow USP SOP for cleaning and gowning.
- Thoroughly wash hands, nails, and arms up to the elbow with antiseptic cleansing agent and water for 30 seconds.
- Dry hands with a non-shedding towel.
- Cover gown must be donned.
- Wear protective gloves.
- Gloves should extend over the gown cuffs.
- Gloves should be sprayed with isopropyl alcohol 70% and rubbed thoroughly.
- Allow gloves to air dry before proceeding with sterile preparations.
- Intermittently sterilize gloves with isopropyl alcohol 70%.
- Change glove when torn, punctured, or contaminated.

Step 4: Prepare your mixing surface and trays.
- Clean off your mixing surface with 70% isopropyl alcohol.
- Then bring out your mixing tray and clean off the rubber tops with 70% isopropyl alcohol and allow the rubber tops to dry before inserting a needle in them.

Step 5: Mix the patient's vial.
- Place needles in appropriate dilutions for mixing the patient vial and verify.
- Pull up 0.2 mL of each appropriate antigen dilution and put into the sterile empty vial.
- Add 1 mL of 50% glycerin (unless using HSA as diluent/preservative).
- Add the appropriate amount of diluent.
- Thoroughly mix the patient's vial.
- Store their vial in the refrigerator between 2 and 8 °C.

29.9 The Next Recipe

Once the patient completes 10 doses from that vial, it is time to create the next vial for the patient. The "recipe" for the next vial follows similar principles to the ones used to create their first vial. Now mix all the antigens one dilution stronger (or "one dilution to the right"). Add 1 mL of 50% glycerin.

Remember that if you have 5 or more concentrates in the vial, you don't need to add additional 50% glycerin.

Diluent will then be added to bring the volume up to 5 mL total.

If HSA is being used as a preservative, remember not to add 1 mL of 50% glycerin.

29.10 Recipe Examples for Mixing the Next Patient Vial

Refer to ▶ Table 29.3 for mixing next vial.

Table 29.3 Examples of escalation SCIT vial prescriptions using different diluents

| Using PNS as diluent with 1 mL of 50% glycerin | | | | Using HSA as diluent | | | |
Antigen	Previous dilution	Volume	"One dilution to the right"	Antigen	Previous dilution	Volume	"One dilution to the right"
Cat	#4	0.20 mL	#3	Cat	#4	0.20 mL	#3
Dog	#2	0.20 mL	#1	Dog	#2	0.20 mL	#1
Oak	Conc	0.20 mL	Conc	Oak	Conc	0.20 mL	Conc
Ragweed	#4	0.20 mL	#3	Ragweed	#4	0.20 mL	#3
Add 50% glycerin		1.0 mL		Add HSA diluent		4.2 mL	
Add diluent		3.2 mL		To make total		5.0 mL	
To make total		5.0 mL					

Abbreviations: HSA, human serum albumin; PNS, phenolated normal saline.

29.11 Shot Administration

Allergy injections are given in a clinic which is prepared to handle any potential allergy urgencies or emergencies (see Chapters 34 and 35 on allergy emergencies). If they are not administered in practitioner's clinic, be sure that the clinic that is administering them is properly prepared with appropriate equipment, supplies, and trained personnel. In addition, a supervising practitioner must be in the office suite when injections are being administered.

Prior to injection, the skin is cleaned with an alcohol pad (or similar). Gloves and appropriate personnel protective apparel are used to draw up the appropriate dose for injection. Then, the posterior aspect of the upper arm is grasped to stabilize and isolate the area for injection, drawing subcutaneous adipose tissue away from any muscle (▶ Fig. 29.1a, b). Injections are given subcutaneously and generally administered in the adipose tissue of the posterior aspect of the upper arm. Needles used for injection are of very small caliber and there should be little to no bleeding.

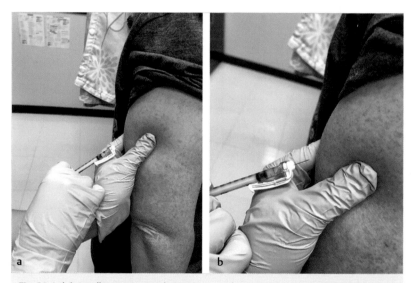

Fig. 29.1 (a) An allergy injection being given in the posterior aspect of the right upper arm. Note the patient's arm is grasped with the nondominant hand to isolate the subcutaneous adipose tissue away from the muscle. **(b)** A close-up of the injection. Note the syringe is all of one piece and the needle is of very small caliber.

Wars have been fought by allergy nurses as to whether or not it is necessary to aspirate prior to injecting for an allergy shot. There is not a lot of evidence either way, however, aspirating before any injection is never a bad idea.

After each injection, the patient should wait in a supervised waiting area for 30 minutes to ensure that there is no adverse reaction prior to leaving this waiting area. Patients on SCIT should also receive a prescription for auto-injectable epinephrine and trained on how to use it.

Some providers practicing immunotherapy, largely otolaryngology allergists, advocate vial testing prior to the first SCIT injection from any newly mixed vial. This is essentially an intradermal test from the newly mixed vial.

29.12 Injection Escalation Protocols

There are a variety of different ways to escalate a patient from the prescribed starting dose of SCIT to the maximum tolerated treatment dose. This is generally done over a 10- to 12-week period, but there are a variety of schedules with alternative dosing/time schemes. In general, shots are given weekly, roughly anywhere between 5 and 10 days apart. ▸ Table 29.4 is an example of one version of an SCIT escalation protocol and ▸ Table 29.5 is an example of a faster SCIT escalation protocol. When first starting an allergy practice, it is strongly advisable to use a slower escalation protocol until the practitioner gains more experience. Faster escalation protocols require careful candidate selection, as they are not appropriate for all patients (i.e., brittle asthmatics, etc.).

Once a patient has reached the determined maintenance dose, injections are generally given weekly for a period of time before spacing the timing of injections further apart. Some practitioners will have patient on weekly injections for 1 year prior to this; others will do weekly injections for 6 months or less, prior to spacing them out. The key is the patient should be experiencing symptomatic relief before any consideration is given to spacing the injections further apart.

29.13 How Much Concentration to Use? What's Considered Therapeutic?

High-dose immunotherapy is generally more efficacious than lower, subtherapeutic doses. Ideally, a patient's vial is escalated until the antigens used in the vial are all taken from concentrate. This would then be considered the patient's maintenance vial prescription; however, select patients may not tolerate that and the treatment dose for those individuals may be held at a weaker dilution.

Table 29.4 Example of an SCIT escalation schedule using weekly injections

	First escalation vial dose	Second escalation vial dose	Third escalation vial dose
Week 1	0.05 mL	0.05 mL	0.05 mL
Week 2	0.1 mL	0.1 mL	0.1 mL
Week 3	0.15 mL	0.15 mL	0.15 mL
Week 4	0.2 mL	0.2 mL	0.2 mL
Week 5	0.25 mL	0.25 mL	0.25 mL
Week 6	0.3 mL	0.3 mL	0.3 mL
Week 7	0.35 mL	0.35 mL	0.35 mL
Week 8	0.4 mL	0.4 mL	0.4 mL
Week 9	0.45 mL	0.45 mL	0.45 mL
Week 10	0.5 mL	0.5 mL	0.5 mL

Abbreviation: SCIT, subcutaneous immunotherapy.
Once patient has reached a vial mixed from concentrates or has reached a determined therapeutic dilution, the patient continues on a dose of 0.5 mL weekly until a determination is made to space out the injections for a longer timeframe or SCIT is stopped.

Table 29.5 Example of a faster SCIT escalation schedule using weekly injections

	First escalation vial dose	Second escalation vial dose	Third escalation vial dose
Week 1	0.05 mL	0.05 mL	0.05 mL
Week 2	0.1 mL	0.1 mL	0.1 mL
Week 3	0.2 mL	0.2 mL	0.2 mL
Week 4	0.3 mL	0.3 mL	0.3 mL
Week 5	0.4 mL	0.4 mL	0.4 mL
Week 6	0.5 mL	0.5 mL	0.5 mL

Abbreviation: SCIT, subcutaneous immunotherapy.
Once patient has reached a vial mixed from concentrates or has reached a determined therapeutic dilution, the patient continues on a dose of 0.5 mL weekly until a determination is made to space out the injections for a longer timeframe or SCIT is stopped.

If a patient begins to complain of very large local reactions (larger than a half dollar in size), which are prolonged in nature, or is beginning to have mild systemic reactions, the escalation of injections should be paused and the patient should be maintained on that dose or a slightly lower, better tolerated dose for a period of time at the discretion of the practitioner. Consideration can be given to trying to advance the patient again in the future to see if the patient can now tolerate a higher dose, but if the patient begins to manifest concerning symptoms again, then that lower dose should likely be considered the thera-peutic dose if it is providing symptom relief.

29.14 What Is the Volume of the Maintenance Injection?

This depends on what protocol a practitioner chooses to use, but may be between 0.5 and 1.0 mL. The examples given in Tables 29.4 and 29.5 use a maintenance volume of 0.5 mL.

29.15 How Long Does a Patient Stay on SCIT? When Do They Stop? Should They Be Retested?

In general, a course of SCIT lasts for 3 to 5 years. Then strong consideration should be given to stopping the course of SCIT, unless special circumstances necessitate continuation of therapy without cessation. Additional testing is *not* necessary to determine if therapy is effective; that determination should be made at the end of the first year of SCIT and assessed by whether that patient is getting symptomatic relief and using fewer medications. If the patient has *not* improved at all on SCIT after 1 year of therapy, *do not* continue. Instead stop SCIT and assess alternative options or investigate (if you have not already done so) the reason as to why the patient has not responded. Additional testing is also not necessary to determine if a patient should stop or continue therapy.

Patients stopping SCIT should be advised to monitor their symptoms for the next 6 months or so. There are some patients who will have a relapse in symptoms in a short period of time who may benefit from restarting SCIT if they wish.

Clinical Pearls   **M!**

- Ensure the vial prescription correlates patient symptoms and test results.
- To reduce volume, use 0.2 mL of the antigen dilution that is 2 dilutions "to the right."
- If PNS is used, be sure to have a total of 1 mL of 50% glycerin in the vial.
- If human serum albumen is used, no extra glycerin is needed to maintain potency.

Bibliography

[1] Cox L, Nelson H, Lockey R, et al. Allergen immunotherapy: a practice parameter third update. J Allergy Clin Immunol. 2011; 127(1) Suppl:S1–S55

30 Immunotherapy: Sublingual Immunotherapy

Bryan Leatherman, Sarah K. Wise, Christine B. Franzese

30.1 Desperately Seeking a Non-Shot Alternative

Many patients are not interested in allergy shots, but would be open to or interested in another form of immunotherapy (IT). Sublingual immunotherapy (SLIT) is a widely practiced allergen IT option that offers an alternative for these patients. Sublingual immunotherapy has demonstrated efficacy in reducing clinical allergy symptoms and medication use. It has an excellent safety profile, although there are some reports of systemic reactions and anaphylaxis; any form of allergen IT requires close patient evaluation, monitoring, and vigilance. Because of its strong safety record, SLIT is usually dosed a home, which provides an additional convenience to patients. Sublingual immunotherapy dosing can be somewhat murky and confusing with respect to actual allergen content, due to differences in published studies and available antigens in different countries and markets.

30.2 Serious Stuff

30.2.1 Why Immunotherapy? Why Sublingual Immunotherapy?

Classic treatment for allergic disease includes avoidance of allergens and/or environmental control measures, pharmacotherapy, and IT. Immunotherapy is the only treatment approach capable of altering the underlying immunopathology of allergy, wherein gradual changes in the body's immune system occur (i.e., shift away from T helper [T_h2] responses, increase in T-regulatory response) such that exposure to the allergen does not elicit substantial clinical symptoms. Immunotherapy can yield long-term symptom reduction even after discontinuing therapy and, in some studies, has been shown to reduce the progression of allergic disease to asthma, as well as the development of new allergen sensitizations. It can reduce a patient's long-term medication requirements and overall health care costs over time.

SCIT has been the predominant method of IT in the United States since it was introduced around 100 years ago. There are certain risks associated with injection IT, such as anaphylactic reactions, that make alternative approaches of IT delivery attractive. In addition, although very rare, deaths have resulted from

SCIT administration. Various alternative methods of allergen IT have been proposed and utilized throughout the years. These include oral IT (swallowing allergen for action/absorption in the gut), bronchial inhalation of allergen, nasal routes of allergen administration, and intraocular IT. However, due to marginal benefit or the provocation of substantial and uncomfortable side effects, these IT methods are not commonly used.

Sublingual immunotherapy is the one alternative IT modality that has been widely adopted throughout the world. It differs from oral IT by holding the antigen under the tongue for a period of time before either spitting it out, or more commonly, swallowing the antigen. The SLIT technique was first introduced in the United States in the 1940s; however, it did not gain widespread use at that time. In recent decades, SLIT administration has substantially increased in the United States.

30.2.2 How Does SLIT Work?

There are dendritic cells in the sublingual mucosa, which are antigen-presenting cells. Allergens contained in the SLIT preparation are taken up directly in the sublingual region. This is why it is important to keep the SLIT aqueous solution or tablet held under the tongue for the requisite amount of time, often 2 minutes. The antigen travels to the lymph node within 12 to 24 hours and is processed in a similar fashion to SCIT. Given frequent exposure to food preparations, medications, etc., it is thought that the immunologic mechanisms of the sublingual mucosa may demonstrate increased tolerance compared to the skin and subcutaneous tissue. This may be one reason for the increased safety profile seen with SLIT. For those interested in the specifics—immune suppressive mediators such as interleukin (IL)-10, transforming growth factor (TGF)-beta, and interferon are constitutively produced in the oral mucosa. Also, the oral tissues contain a relatively low number of proinflammatory cells such as eosinophils and macrophages.

30.2.3 What Evidence Do We Have for SLIT Efficacy?

In the mid-1980s, the first "modern" studies of SLIT were reported. Since that time, numerous investigators, mostly from European centers, have described the clinical efficacy and basic science of SLIT. In 1998, the World Health Organization reported that there was sufficient efficacy and safety data available to conclude that SLIT was an acceptable means of IT administration. A subsequent publication by the European Academy of Allergy and Clinical Immunology, as well as the Allergic Rhinitis and its Impact on Asthma (ARIA) document agreed with the utility of SLIT in adults and children.

Presently, in adults, SLIT is considered moderately efficacious for the treatment of allergic rhinitis/rhinoconjunctivitis when compared to placebo, based on several systematic reviews and meta-analyses. With longer treatment, SLIT is considered highly efficacious. In clinical trials, the benefit of SLIT is seen over and above symptom benefit obtained from the use of rescue medications. For children, the strength of SLIT evidence appears to vary by allergen, based on current data. The efficacy of grass pollen SLIT in children is supported by strong evidence, while there is moderate-to-low quality evidence to support house dust mite SLIT in children at the present time.

There are very few head-to-head studies of SLIT versus SCIT, and in most of these, the sample size is small. Meta-analyses-based indirect comparisons of SLIT and SCIT have been performed recently, with some publications reporting that SCIT is more efficacious than SLIT, although this evidence is considered weak at this time.

There have been some investigations into the efficacy of SLIT in preventing the development of asthma and new allergen sensitizations. Although the results of some trials are promising, the strength of evidence is considered to be relatively low overall. Additional investigation into the "preventative effects" of SLIT would be helpful to improve the overall understanding of SLIT efficacy.

30.2.4 SLIT Is Safer Than SCIT. True or False?

Sublingual immunotherapy is generally considered safer than SCIT. This improved safety profile allows for home administration of SLIT, which is more convenient for patients. For patients who are not able to make regular clinic visits for injections, home administration makes IT feasible.

In order to fully understand the safety profile of SLIT, it is best to compare it to SCIT. In a recent survey report of the American Academy of Allergy, Asthma and Immunology and the American College of Allergy, Asthma, and Immunology between 2008 and 2013, 28.9 million injection visits were analyzed. There was a systemic reaction rate of 0.1% of injection visits, with grade 4 systemic reactions reported at 0.1 per 10,000 injections. There were two fatalities that occurred during SCIT under the care of allergists and two fatalities that occurred under the care of non-allergists. While anaphylaxis and deaths have been reported with SCIT, it is important to note that the rate of serious events is very low, and with proper screening and precautions in place, SCIT is a very safe form of IT.

The first report of anaphylaxis with SLIT was published in 2006, and since that time, there have been several case reports that followed. In 2012, an analysis of the rate of anaphylaxis during SLIT was published, noting one case of anaphylaxis per 100 million SLIT doses, or one case of anaphylaxis per 526,000 SLIT treatment years. This is exceptionally low. To authors' knowledge, there have been no deaths reported with SLIT. Based upon the published rates of systemic reaction and anaphylaxis, SLIT is generally accepted as having a higher safety profile than SCIT.

30.2.5 What Is the Best Dose of SLIT to Give to Patients?

The optimal dosage, timing of administration, and optimal length of treatment with SLIT are not clearly defined. The majority of modern dosing information available in the literature comes from European studies utilizing antigens that are not available in the United States. It is difficult to directly translate the antigen content of sublingual preparations utilized in the majority of the published European studies into dosing with United States allergens. Therefore, it can be difficult to establish the effective dose of SLIT utilizing the liquid-based antigen preparations available in the United States. However, one fairly consistent finding is that higher doses of antigen are generally necessary for SLIT compared to SCIT. It is also clear that SLIT is safe over a wide dosing range.

In 2015, Leatherman and colleagues thoroughly examined the available literature with regard to SLIT dosing. Evidence available at that time revealed that SLIT dosing ranges (in µg/day) could be recommended for *Dermatophagoides pteronyssinus*, *D. farinae*, timothy grass, Bermuda grass, ragweed, and "other" pollen. At that time, all other allergens did not have sufficient evidence to recommend SLIT dose ranges. In order to aid the practitioner, some recommended ranges of allergen concentrates to add to aqueous SLIT vials were given. This is a helpful guide to understand the current evidence on SLIT dosing.

The appropriate timing and duration of SLIT have not been defined. In various clinical trials, the antigen has been delivered perennially, preseasonal/coseasonal, as well as coseasonal alone. It is generally accepted that perennial administration of SCIT for 3 to 5 years is preferable to achieve long-term maintenance of the improvement after IT has been completed. For SLIT, however, benefit has been shown with perennial administration, variations of preseasonal/coseasonal administration, and even alternating (months on/months off) administration. Thus, there may be multiple options available for SLIT dosing that can be tailored to the needs of individual patients. These different treatment options will have to be clarified by future trials.

30.2.6 Now Let's Get Practical. How to Do This?

As discussed, there are various options for SLIT administration. Options also exist regarding the specific product type. Currently SLIT tablets are available in the United States for grass pollen, ragweed, and house dust mite. Alternatively, may practitioners choose off-label use of aqueous antigens, typically administered in multiple-allergen mixes. In truth, this is one of the areas in need of the most research in the SLIT arena. We have very little data on the efficacy of multiple-allergen SLIT mixes, yet this is a commonly practiced treatment in the United States. For aqueous SLIT mixes, many practitioners mix their own vials in their offices. There are also third-party pharmacies that will mix vials as well.

Sublingual immunotherapy tablets are approved by the Food and Drug Administration (FDA). There are specific indications and contraindications on the package labeling, along with dosing instructions. It is recommended that the first dose be given in the physician's office, and a prescription for an epinephrine auto-injector is required.

For aqueous SLIT administration, consider the following:

- Patient education is key. The following are some important points for education:
  - How to dose the drops (i.e., dose and count the drops while looking in the mirror, hold under the tongue for 2 minutes, then swallow).
  - Side effects of SLIT (i.e., oral cavity itching, gastrointestinal upset).
  - Signs of anaphylaxis.
- Prescription for epinephrine self-injector.
- Presence of a parent when drops are given to children.
- Administration of first dose in the clinic (strongly recommended).

As with any form of IT, clinical follow-up of SLIT patients is necessary. Most practitioners see patients every 6 months, although this may vary by practice and individual patient needs. Validated questionnaires are very helpful to monitor symptoms and medication use.

30.2.7 How to Mix an Aqueous SLIT Vial

One method to mix an aqueous SLIT vial uses a two-stage process where a maintenance vial is mixed first, then an escalation vial is made from that maintenance vial. To mix the maintenance vial, use 1 mL of antigen concentrate for each positive allergen that should be treated, generally up to a total of 10 antigens. Why 10 antigens? Mainly because 10 mL vials are frequently used and with 1 mL per antigen is the maximum number of antigens that would fit in the vial. If less than 10 antigens are used, then 50% glycerin is used as the diluent to bring the total amount of liquid in the vial to 10 mL. See ▶ Table 30.1 for example of mixing SLIT vial.

If you happen to use endpoints to mix your SCIT recipes, do not do that for SLIT method. Note that no endpoint is needed as antigen concentrate is used to mix these types of vials.

Table 30.1 Sublingual immunotherapy **maintenance vial**

Antigen	Volume
Cat	1.0 mL concentrate
Dog	1.0 mL concentrate
Oak	1.0 mL concentrate
Ragweed	1.0 mL concentrate
Add diluent (50% glycerin)	6.0 mL
To make total	10.0 mL

Once this vial is completed, the escalation vial can be mixed but note that this vial will only be used once for a short time and then discarded. Once the escalation vial is completed, all further treatment will come from the maintenance vial and all future vials will be mixed according to that recipe. There will be no need to make additional escalation vials in the future.

To mix the escalation vial, 0.25 mL is taken from the newly created maintenance vial and added to a separate (usually smaller) vial. Then add 1 mL of 50% glycerin to complete the creation of the escalation vial. See ▶ Table 30.2 for escalation vial.

Be sure to clearly label each vial. Since the patient will be administering the bulk of the SLIT doses from these vials at home, it is very helpful to use different color labels for each vial and give the patient specific instructions on how to perform the escalation and when to discard the escalation vial.

So there's a lot we don't know about aqueous SLIT, but if I decide to do this, what kind of vials might be used for this? And how could it be dosed?

Table 30.2 Sublingual immunotherapy **escalation vial**

Antigen	Volume
Maintenance vial	0.25 mL
Add diluent (50% glycerin)	1.0 mL
To make total	1.25 mL

► Fig. 30.1 shows different types of vials. How SLIT is dosed will depend on what type of vial is used. Some allergists will use a dropper vial and use a dosing protocol that reaches a maintenance dose of five drops per day, while others will use three or seven drops. Some may use a vial with a pump style dispenser and may use a dosing protocol that reaches a maintenance dose of two to five pumps, depending on what volume of SLIT is desired daily by the allergist and how much liquid is dispensed with each pump. Some will use a screw top vial and a small needleless tuberculin (TB) or insulin syringe for administration. The patient needs to unscrew the vial and use the syringe to draw up an exact amount of liquid to place under the tongue.

It is helpful to have the patient take the first dose of SLIT in the office, not only to see if they tolerate it, but also to ensure that the patient is taking it correctly. This is especially important if using a dropper vial. To properly administer a dose with a dropper vial, patients should watch themselves in a mirror and count the drops. However, not infrequently, patients will be convinced that they can "feel" the drops and not use a mirror to dispense the correct dose. In actuality, a single drop is usually too small an amount for a patient to feel it and most often multiple drops are dispensed before the patient "feels" (and counts) one drop. This will lead to overdosing and the vial will run out much faster than it should.

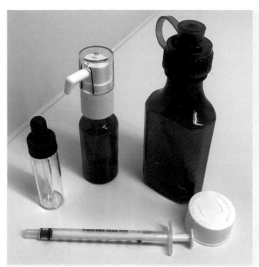

Fig. 30.1 Different types of vials.

See ▶ Table 30.3 for one example of an escalation and maintenance dosing protocol using a dropper vial method. ▶ Table 30.4 is an example of a combined dropper vial/syringe dosing protocol.

Table 30.3 Example of a dropper-vial based escalation and maintenance dosing protocol

Number of drops from escalation vial	
Day 1	1 drop
Day 2	2 drops
Day 3	3 drops
Day 4	4 drops
Day 5	5 drops

Discard escalation vial, continue with drops from maintenance vial

Number of drops from maintenance vial	
Day 6	1 drop
Day 7	2 drops
Day 8	3 drops
Day 9	4 drops
Day 10	5 drops
Day 11 and on	Continue using 5 drops daily

Table 30.4 Example of a dropper/syringe-based escalation and maintenance dosing protocol

Number of drops from escalation vial	
Day 1	1 drop
Day 2	2 drops
Day 3	3 drops
Day 4	4 drops
Day 5	5 drops

Discard escalation vial, continue with drops from maintenance vial

Amount from maintenance vial	
Day 6	0.1 mL
Day 7	0.1 mL
Day 8	0.2 mL
Day 9	Continue taking 0.2 mL daily

30.2.8 How Long Do These Maintenance Vials Last? Do They Need to Be Refrigerated?

Exactly how long the 10-mL vials last will depend on the specific dosing proto-col but generally will last between 12 and 16 weeks. Generally, these vials do not need to be refrigerated, although some practitioners do recommend refrig-erating them. Patients should be advised not to freeze these vials, leave them in direct sunlight, in the glove compartment of a car, or other place that may be subject to temperature extremes.

30.2.9 What *Don't* We Know About SLIT?

In the past two decades, the published evidence relating to SLIT has grown immensely. However, there are still some unanswered questions. These are just a few of the items that should be addressed in future studies:

- What is the magnitude of SLIT efficacy compared to SCIT? Large head-to-head studies are needed.
- Is multi-allergen therapy with SLIT efficacious?
- What are the best dosing and escalation regimens for SLIT?
  - How can safety and efficacy be maximized with SLIT dosing?
  - Are dosing and escalation regimens antigen-dependent?
  - Preseasonal, coseasonal, or continuous administration—does it really matter?
- Can SLIT really prevent the progression to asthma or new allergen sensitivities?

| Clinical Pearls | **M!** |

- SLIT is efficacious in reducing clinical allergy symptoms and medication use.
- SLIT has a high safety profile, but the practitioner should be aware of the possibility of systemic reactions including anaphylaxis.
- SLIT is usually dosed a home, which is a valued convenience for patients.
- There is some evidence available to support SLIT dosing ranges for certain antigens, although additional research is needed in this area.

Bibliography

[1] Anonymous. Allergen immunotherapy: therapeutic vaccines for allergic diseases. Geneva: January 27–29 1997. Allergy. 1998; 53(44) Suppl:1–42

[2] Calderón MA, Simons FE, Malling HJ, Lockey RF, Moingeon P, Demoly P. Sublingual allergen immunotherapy: mode of action and its relationship with the safety profile. Allergy. 2012; 67(3):302–311

[3] Cox LS, Larenas Linnemann D, Nolte H, Weldon D, Finegold I, Nelson HS. Sublingual immunotherapy: a comprehensive review. J Allergy Clin Immunol. 2006; 117(5):1021–1035

[4] Epstein TG, Liss GM, Murphy-Berendts K, Bernstein DI. Risk factors for fatal and nonfatal reactions to subcutaneous immunotherapy: National surveillance study on allergen immunotherapy (2008–2013). Ann Allergy Asthma Immunol. 2016; 116(4):354–359.e2

[5] Hankin CS, Cox L, Lang D, et al. Allergen immunotherapy and health care cost benefits for children with allergic rhinitis: a large-scale, retrospective, matched cohort study. Ann Allergy Asthma Immunol. 2010; 104(1):79–85

[6] Hankin CS, Cox L, Lang D, et al. Allergy immunotherapy among Medicaid-enrolled children with allergic rhinitis: patterns of care, resource use, and costs. J Allergy Clin Immunol. 2008; 121(1):227–232

[7] Leatherman BD, Khalid A, Lee S, et al. Dosing of sublingual immunotherapy for allergic rhinitis: evidence-based review with recommendations. Int Forum Allergy Rhinol. 2015; 5(9):773–783

[8] Malling H, Abreu-Noguera J, Alvarez-Cuesta E, et al. EAACI/ESPACI position paper on local immunotherapy. Allergy. 1998; 53:833–844

[9] Wise SK, Lin SY, Toskala E, et al. International Consensus Statement on Allergy and Rhinology: Allergic Rhinitis. Int Forum Allergy Rhinol. 2018; 8(2):108–352

159

31 Sublingual Tablets

Christine B. Franzese

31.1 Looking for Unicorns

"I've never seen a patient only allergic to one thing. Why would you ever use (insert name of sublingual immunotherapy [SLIT] tablet here)?" The author uses sublingual tablets, however, this question is posed by many patients. Particularly in the United States, where the population is predominately polysensitized, finding a symptomatic monosensitized patient in an allergy clinic is probably like finding a unicorn, just not as exciting. The good news is that, while these tablets are great options for monosensitized patients, they work just as well for symptomatic relief in polysensitized patients. In fact, studies done for these tablets to obtain Food and Drug Administration (FDA) approval included polysensitized patients. While these tablets may not be the best option for all allergy patients, neither are shots. However, these tablets may be very good options for most of the patients and may even help bring in new patients to an allergy practice.

31.2 Who Is a Candidate for Sublingual Immunotherapy Tablet?

Anyone can be a candidate for immunotherapy. Anyone who has symptoms of allergic disease, positive allergy testing that correlates to their symptoms, does not have medical comorbidities which would reduce the chance of survival in the event of anaphylaxis, is not pregnant at initiation, does not have uncontrolled or poorly controlled asthma, and is not on any medications which would complicate treatment in the event of anaphylaxis. In addition, SLIT tablets should not be used in patients with eosinophilic esophagitis.

31.3 The Practical Applications of Tablets

There are groups of patients for whom tablet therapy works well. The following are examples of types of polysensitized patients where a SLIT tablet could be used:

- **"Fallen off the bandwagon" (FotB):** Subcutaneous immunotherapy (SCIT) injection patients who have stopped coming in for their injections prior to completing a course of treatment. There's a host of reasons why patients stop coming for injections, but regardless—if they have a history of symptoms and a positive test result to an antigen in one of the SLIT tablets, they are a candidate for this therapy. It may even help bring some of these patients back into the clinic. This has been discussed at the end of the chapter.

- **"Not able to do SCIT, can't afford SLIT":** Some patients may not be able to fit weekly injections into their lifestyles for a multitude of reasons. In addition, many insurance companies don't cover (non-tablet) SLIT, and some patients can't afford the out-of-pocket costs. These tablets are generally covered under patients' pharmacy benefits, can be done at home, and while the SLIT tablets may not cover all of patients' relevant allergens, patients can still receive the benefits of immunotherapy by using them.

- **"Not here for 5":** The course of immunotherapy is generally 5 years. While no one can predict with certainty that they'll be in a certain area for at least 5 years, some patients know for sure they won't—military personnel, college students, some businesspersons, TV/print journalists, etc. These are just a few examples of patient groups that may move frequently or only be in particular location for a short time. However, that doesn't mean they're not candidates for immunotherapy. Sublingual immunotherapy tablets are easy to travel with and can be obtained nationwide. As long as it is anticipated that the patient will be in areas of the United States or in the world where the antigen that the SLIT tablet is treating is present in, then using a tablet is appropriate.

- **"The peaked polysensitized":** Polysensitized patients who either complain of symptoms in one season or have very mild symptoms at other times of the year, but have one season that causes them real problems. These patients are good candidate for ragweed or timothy grass SLIT tablets, if they have corresponding symptoms for the respective seasons and positive testing.

- **"The peakless polysensitized":** Polysensitized patients who complain of year-round symptoms either with no seasonal peaks, or very mild season symptoms. If significantly sensitized/symptomatic to house dust mites (HDM), these patients are good candidates for HDM tablet therapy.

31.4 SLIT Tablets (Available in the United States)

There are currently four SLIT tablets commercially available for use in the United States. Each will be discussed briefly by antigen. A summary of things common to all four tablets are given as follows.

31.4.1 Timothy Grass

- **Timothy grass pollen allergen extract tablet (Grastek):** For ages from 5 to 65 with symptoms of allergic rhinitis/conjunctivitis during grass season and positive allergy tests to timothy grass or a timothy grass family member;

may be used preseasonally/coseasonally starting about 12 weeks prior to season start or year-round for 3 years for sustained effect.

○ **Dose:** One tablet daily (2,800 bioequivalent allergy units [BAU])

- **Sweet vernal, Orchard, perennial rye, timothy, and Kentucky blue grass mixed pollens allergy extract (Oralair):** Also known as "the five grass tablet." For ages 10 to 65 with symptoms of allergic rhinitis/conjunctivitis during grass season and positive allergy tests to timothy grass or a timothy grass family member. Used preseasonally/coseasonally, starting about 16 weeks prior to season start.

○ **Dose:** One tablet daily for 18 years and above (300 index of reactivity [IR]). For 10–17 years, one 100 IR tablet on day 1; two 100 IR tablets on day 2; and one 300 IR tablet thereafter.

In essence, for timothy grass family member allergies both of these two tablets can be used. However, one meta-analysis demonstrated superiority of the five-grass tablet over the timothy grass tablet.

31.4.2 Ragweed

- **Short ragweed pollen allergen extract tablet (Ragwitek):** For ages 18 to 65 years with symptoms of allergic rhinitis/conjunctivitis during ragweed season and positive allergy tests to ragweed (short, giant, etc.); may be used preseasonally/coseasonally starting about 12 weeks before the start of season.

○ **Dose:** One tablet daily (12 Amb a 1-Unit [Amb a 1-U])

31.4.3 House Dust Mite

- **House dust mite (*Dermatophagoides farinae* and *D. pteronyssinus*) allergy extract tablet (Odactra):** For ages 18 to 65 years with symptoms of year-round allergic rhinitis/conjunctivitis and positive allergy tests to one or both dust mite species in the tablet. Can be initiated at any point in the year.

○ **Dose:** One tablet daily (12 SQ-HDM)

31.4.4 Common to All SLIT Tablets

- Follow the instructions for use for each particular tablet.

> Prior to initiation in the office, do not send patients home with a starter pack or mail the starter pack to their house.

- **Must be initiated in the office:** Patients must take the first tablet in the office and wait for 30 minutes afterward to ensure they do not have any adverse reactions. If no problems at initiation, patients may take all subsequent tablets at home.

> Have your allergy staff instruct patients on how to take these tablets and have the patients demonstrate this back to the nurses with their first dose. Be sure to instruct patients to wash their hands before and after handling the tablets. The tablets disintegrate easily and tablet particles can remain on patients' hands.

- "On Label" use requires that a form of auto-injectable epinephrine is prescribed to the patient.
- Patients should not eat or drink 5 to 10 minutes before or after administration.
- Some patients will have mild local reactions/side effects. These are self-limited, usually last no more than 15 minutes, and cause no loss of speech/swallowing.

These side effects are similar to what you would expect to a patient receiving an allergy shot. Many patients will have some mild swelling, redness, and itching/irritation at their injection site. A similar phenomenon can occur for a few weeks with the SLIT tablets. Using an antihistamine of patient's choice daily for about a month helps limit this.

- Patients with worsening symptoms/side effects, such as tongue swelling, should discontinue therapy.
- Patients should call and discontinue therapy if symptoms of potential eosinophilic esophagitis occur (severe/persistent reflux symptoms despite treatment).
- Patients should call and discontinue therapy prior to any oral surgery/dental extractions or if any oral ulcers/open wounds. Once healed, most patients can restart therapy.

31.5 Tablet Cannibalism and Bringing in New Patients to the Practice

Another major concern about SLIT tablets is that they might "cannibalize" your SCIT practice, meaning, they will not add new patients to your practice and will draw potential shot patients away from SCIT thus decreasing your revenue. This doesn't seem to occur in actual practice.

The author has witnessed that there are a significant number of patients who, regardless of symptom severity, do not want shots and will not seek the care of an allergist or get allergy testing because going to an allergist is equivalent to getting shots. This group of patients would never normally seek the care of an allergist, but when hearing about non-shot options, they become interested in immunotherapy. This is similar to the effect that "sinus balloons" or balloon Sinuplasty has had on sinus surgery in otolaryngology practices. Balloon Sinuplasty is somewhat controversial, but regardless of which side of the sinus balloon debate has been chosen, this procedure is attractive to patients who never would have considered sinus surgery prior to this. While the author performs this procedure rarely, often a patient says something to the effect of "I have terrible sinus problems but never got checked out because I had a brother/sister/(insert relative here) who had sinus surgery in the past and it was the worst experience ever. But…I heard about this sinus balloon thing…." A similar phenomenon occurs with SLIT tablet usage: Patients who would otherwise never darken your door find out about a non-shot option and come to explore treatment options.

Clinical Pearls M!

- First tablet must be taken in the office and patient must wait for 30 minutes afterward.
- Criteria to be a candidate is similar to SCIT.
- "On-label" use requires a prescription for an epinephrine pen.
- Consider using this in your practice. You may be surprised to find a place for them and that they help build your patient base.

Bibliography

[1] Devillier P, Dreyfus JF, Demoly P, Calderón MA. A meta-analysis of sublingual allergen immunotherapy and pharmacotherapy in pollen-induced seasonal allergic rhinoconjunctivitis. BMC Med. 2014; 12:71

[2] Wise SK, Lin SY, Toskala E, et al. International Consensus Statement on Allergy and Rhinology: Allergic Rhinitis. Int Forum Allergy Rhinol. 2018; 8(2):108–352

32 Oral Mucosal Immunotherapy

Christine B. Franzese

32.1 Becoming Part of the Routine

One major factor in successful immunotherapy is patient compliance. Regardless of how well subcutaneous immunotherapy (SCIT) works, if the patient doesn't come to receive their injections then SCIT will not work for that patient. Similarly with aqueous sublingual immunotherapy (SLIT) drops, if the patient doesn't take the drops as directed then SLIT will not work for them. Incorporating patients' allergy treatment in their daily routine may make it easier for them to be compliant with therapy. Take allergy toothpaste, for example. Most people brush their teeth every day as part of their routine, and recommendations are to do so for 2 minutes—the same amount of time a patient has to hold aqueous SLIT drops under their tongue. Why not take advantage of that?

32.2 Allergy Toothpaste—Say What?

Oral mucosal immunotherapy (OMIT) is a different way to deliver antigen to the immune system using a glycerin-based toothpaste vehicle that does not contain fluoride. It involves taking advantage of the density and characteristics of oral Langerhans cells. Langerhans cells in the oral cavity possess high affinity immunoglobulin E (IgE) receptors, are able to bind and present processed antigens to local T-cells, and induce an inhibitory T-helper (T_h2) response. While both SLIT and OMIT use these cells, it has been discovered that the sublingual mucosa (where SLIT is placed) has the lowest density and buccal and vestibular region (of which OMIT takes advantage) have the highest density of these cells.

32.3 A Word Before We Start

This is a relatively new allergy therapy that does not have much literature behind it yet, but is currently under further investigation. There are a few studies in the literature that demonstrate its effectiveness, but it has not been studied nearly as extensively as SCIT or SLIT. However, it is currently being used in practice. If a practitioner chooses to use this therapy as part of their treatment, they should make sure to advise patients that, similar to SLIT drops, OMIT is not covered by insurance and the patient has to bear the expenses.

32.4 Who Is a Candidate for OMIT?

Anyone who brushes his/her teeth at least once a day is candidate for OMIT. As discussed in the immediately preceding chapters, anyone who has symptoms of allergic disease, has positive allergy testing that correlates to their symptoms, does not have medical comorbidities which would reduce the chance of survival in the event of anaphylaxis, is not pregnant at initiation, does not have uncontrolled or poorly controlled asthma, and is not on any medications which would complicate treatment in the event of anaphylaxis.

32.5 How to Mix Oral Mucosal Immunotherapy

Oral mucosal immunotherapy toothpaste comes in a kit containing toothpaste base to which antigen is added, a toothpaste dispenser to which the mixed allergen-containing toothpaste is added, then assembled, and additional supplies for mixing, such as sterile tongue depressors (▶ Fig. 32.1). Mixing of the paste should occur in the same area where other vials are mixed, in a USP 797-compliant area by appropriately trained staff after the designated area has been cleaned per protocol.

In general, the toothpaste is compatible with glycerinated antigens and will hold a total of 20 mL of glycerinated antigen plus any needed diluent. To mix, 2 mL of each antigen that is desired to be used for treatment is added to the toothpaste base, accommodating a maximum of 10 antigens. If fewer than 10 antigens are used, enough glycerin is added to bring the total volume up to

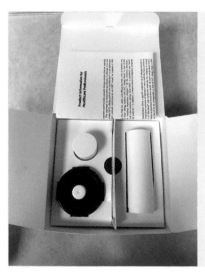

Fig. 32.1 The contents of an OMIT kit.

20 mL. If there is a desire to treat with more than 10 antigens, a decision must be made as to whether less than 2 mL per antigen are used or mix 2 tubes of toothpaste.

32.6 How to Use Oral Mucosal Immunotherapy

Typically, most people brush their teeth twice a day and OMIT is also dosed twice daily, using one pump of the toothpaste dispenser (▶ Fig. 32.2). The patients must brush their teeth for 2 minutes, which is what dentists recommend. It can be helpful for patients to get musical toothbrushes that play a song for 2 minutes or toothbrushes that light up for 2 minutes or have some method of timing their brushing. If the patient only brushes once a day, the dosing can be altered to two pumps once a day.

This toothpaste doesn't contain fluoride. If a high-risk dental patient is being treated who needs fluoride, then either a request can be made to a compounding company to add fluoride to the toothpaste base (which the author do not recommend because it would be expensive method) or dosing can be adjusted to once daily, so that the allergen toothpaste is used at one time and the fluoride prescription toothpaste needed by the high-risk dental patient is used the other times during the day (author recommends this as it is much less expensive method).

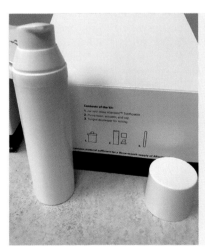

Fig. 32.2 The pasted is mixed, then placed into a toothpaste dispenser pump.

The patient should brush their teeth in clinic with the allergy toothpaste the first time they use it and then wait for 30 minutes to ensure they can tolerate it without adverse event. Side effects and adverse events are similar to those seen with SLIT. Giving the patient a prescription for auto-injectable epinephrine is left to the providers' discretion.

The toothpaste base comes in two flavors at present, mint and berry (▶ Fig. 32.3). While my practice carries both flavors, by far the mint flavor is the most popular, even with young children. If first starting out using OMIT, stocking more of the mint flavor at first is recommended.

Patients are generally monitored for compliance and response every 6 months for the first year. If there is no improvement in symptoms, OMIT should be discontinued and the treatment plan be reassessed as done with any immunotherapy nonresponder. If the patient has significant symptom improvement, then the patient should be monitored on an annual basis for 3 to 5 years, or until therapy is discontinued.

32.7 A Word Before We End

The author uses OMIT in personal allergy practice and find it both useful and effective. However, at the beginning of an allergy practice, using OMIT is generally not recommended. The physician should acquire more experience before using OMIT. The author finds OMIT very useful in a certain select populations—anyone who would be a SCIT or SLIT candidate, but where compliance may be an issue due to busyness or forgetfulness (some working adults) or due to inability to perform the mechanics of SLIT drops (i.e., holding the SLIT drops under the tongue for 2 minutes), such as young children.

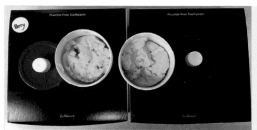

Fig. 32.3 The toothpaste base comes in 2 different flavors, mint and berry, which are identical in color, but smell very different.

Clinical Pearls	M!

- This is a different antigen delivery system, using glycerinated toothpaste base with no fluoride.
- A criterion to be a candidate is similar to SCIT/SLIT.
- Auto-infectible epinephrine is prescribed at the discretion of the provider.
- Mixed using 2 mL per glycerinated antigen for a total of 20 mL of glycerinated antigen plus any diluent.
- For the first use have the patient brush teeth with paste for 2 minutes in the office and wait for 30 minutes afterward.
- Dosing is one pump for twice a day brushing; two pumps for once a day brushing.

Bibliography

[1] Reisacher W, Rudner S, Kotik V. Oral mucosal immunotherapy using a toothpaste delivery system for the treatment of allergic rhinitis. Int J Pharm Compd. 2014; 18(4):287–290

[2] Reisacher WR, Suurna MV, Rochlin K, Bremberg MG, Tropper G. Oral mucosal immunotherapy for allergic rhinitis: a pilot study. Allergy Rhinol (Providence). 2016; 7(1):21–28

33 Treatment: Monosensitization Versus Polysensitization

Christine B. Franzese

33.1 The Eternal Question

To treat or not to treat? That is the question every practitioner faces when selecting antigens to place into the patient's immunotherapy vial. As discussed in Chapter 3, there is a clinical difference between polysensitization and poly-allergy. Do every single allergen that tested positive be treated? Only one or a few antigens are needed—based on the patient's symptoms or the test results or potency of the antigen or some other criteria? This question is quite controversial and how it is answered can be influenced by geographic location, current knowledge, and provider attitudes/confidence/beliefs. Whether this question is consciously addressed or not by the clinician, it's one that must be reconciled each and every time a vial prescription is created.

33.2 Treating the Monosensitized/Monoallergic and the Paucisensitized/Pauciallergic Patient

Treating these types of patients, at first glance, seems simple. Some would argue treating this type of patient is easy because this type of patient doesn't exist. That's not actually true. While the prevalence of mono/paucisensitization versus polysensitization patients varies geographically, mono/paucisensitized patients are present everywhere in the world. These patients may be less likely to seek treatment because the allergens they are allergic to are avoidable or controlled well with medication. Regardless, physician may encounter patients who fall into this category and there are some treatment questions that need to be reconciled.

Do they have enough "allergies" to "need" treatment? The author's allergy nurses ask this question or some variant of it from time to time after testing a patient—"Is that patient allergic 'enough' to get shots? Are they positive to 'enough' allergens?" When creating a treatment plan, this is the wrong question to ask. Patient treatment should be individualized and the decision as to whether or not to treat should be based on patient symptomology, lack of symptom control by medication(s), and/or patient's desire for treatment, not just test results. It should never be based solely on a number—whether that number is the number of positive test results, the size of a skin wheal, or some other arbitrary number.

Can't these patients be treated with medication? Of course. Any patient can be treated, including polysensitized patients, with medication alone. The more important questions to answer are "Is this medication(s) controlling that patient's symptoms without significant side effects," and "Is this how the patient desires to be treated?"

These patients may be great candidates for sublingual tablet therapy.

33.3 Treating the Polysensitized/Polyallergic Patient: Mono/Pauci Therapy

This type of patient can pose more of a challenge, particularly when choosing to treat with mono/pauci therapy. How to select the right antigens? How many of those are to be treated? It is helpful to remember the discussion in Chapter 3 does not equal allergy. Matching patient symptoms to positive test results can be helpful in selecting the correct antigen(s), but there is the potential that history alone may not reveal all important exposures. Cross-reactivity and sensitization to panallergens must also be taken into account when treating the polysensitized patient. Cross-reactivity occurs when immunoglobulin E (IgE) antibodies react with structurally similar allergens in closely related species, such as birch and alder or cottonwood and aspen. Panallergens are thought to be families of related proteins involved in overall vital processes and widely distributed throughout nature. Due to the highly conserved sequence regions and structures of these proteins, they can demonstrate cross-reactivity despite being from unrelated organisms.

There is evidence that using monotherapy improves allergic symptoms in the polysensitized/polyallergic patient. The efficacy of grass, ragweed, and house dust mite-SLIT-tablets in monsensitized and polysensitized patients has been examined and no reduction in efficacy has been found in polysensitized patients in any of these studies. The Polysensitization Impact On Allergan Immunotherapy (POLISMAIL) studies took place in a more real-life setting, in a series of multicenter, observational studies to examine the clinical impact of polysensitizations. The POLISMAIL series demonstrated that immunotherapy with one or two allergen extracts can achieve significant improvement in polysensitized patients.

33.4 Treating the Polysensitized/Polyallergic Patient: Polytherapy

Polytherapy is very popular in the United States and certainly, treating the polysensitized patient with polytherapy seems easier. This therapy seems reassuring to the clinician (and the patient) that "nothing is being missed" and that the patient is being treated with everything relevant. It is not always easy to uncover all relevant exposures from the patient and, although component resolved testing may be helpful in teasing out cross-reactivity or panallergen sensitization in the future, its current utility in clinical practice has yet to be established. Also, vial size is not infinite and in a patient with a great number of sensitivities, the practitioner may still face the dilemma of what doesn't go in the vial. Antigen mixes may be used, but this raises concerns over what exactly is being treated, and are relevant antigens being diluted out by lesser or nonrelevant antigens.

In addition, there is lack of good evidence supporting the efficacy of polytherapy or its superiority to mono/paucitherapy in polysensitized patients. Certainly, the cost of doing a high-quality, randomized, controlled, multi-institutional trial comparing mono/paucitherapy to polytherapy would be enormous, let alone very complicated, which is likely why such evidence is lacking. If a practitioner chooses to practice polytherapy, he/she should reconcile to this fact: there is lack of published clinical evidence to support what is being done. Still, in the United States, most allergy providers practice polytherapy.

33.5 Financial Implications

The author encourages practitioners to calculate the cost of injection vials or sublingual vials beforehand. Majority of the allergy practitioners have never done this exercise. Antigens are expensive and the cost seems to steadily increase every year. The number of antigens placed in a treatment vial directly impacts the cost of each vial and practitioner's profitability. Particularly for polytherapy practitioners, the more antigens in a treatment vial, the more expensive that vial is to produce; the profit is less from each vial. Conversely for the same price, the fewer antigens in the vial, the more profitable it is.

Of course, patient treatment decisions should not be based off the cost of a particular vial, but this does have relevance to the financial health of practitioner's medical practice and he/she should at least be aware about the cost. Knowing the costs of each vial may help the practitioner curb their desire to put every positive antigens into a patient's vial.

Calculating the cost of a SCIT or SLIT vial may seem intimidating at first if you've never done it before. Keep it simple. Take the total costs for antigens and divide that by the number of antigens you use to get a rough per antigen estimate. Then do the same for diluent and vials. Add these up being sure to take into account how many antigens you add to a vial to get an estimate of what a SCIT/SLIT vial costs you.

Clinical Pearls   M!

- Base treatment decisions for immunotherapy on symptoms, not numbers.
- Mono/pauci therapy works in polysensitized patients.
- Know the cost of your treatment vials. More antigens, more expense.

Bibliography

[1] Ciprandi G, Incorvaia C, Puccinelli P, Scurati S, Masieri S, Frati F. The POLISMAIL lesson: sublingual immunotherapy may be prescribed also in polysensitized patients. Int J Immunopathol Pharmacol. 2010; 23(2):637–640

[2] Damask C. Immunotherapy: Treating with Fewer Allergens? Otolaryngol Clin North Am. 2017; 50 (6):1153–1165

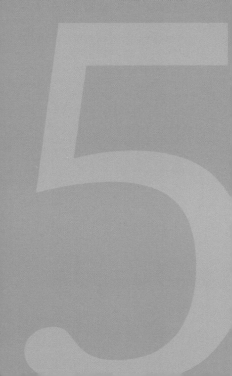

Part 5
Allergy Emergencies

34 Anaphylaxis

Christine B. Franzese

34.1 Keep Calm and Give Epinephrine

Most of the time, an allergy practice runs smoothly with few issues. At some point though, a patient will experience anaphylaxis in the office. Long periods of calm hours are the norm, but these will be abruptly interrupted by a patient having a serious, possibly life-threatening, allergic reaction. So take these words of advice to heart: preparation is the key to treating anaphylaxis. Have an anaphylactic protocol posted at key places in the office. Post sign/symptoms of anaphylaxis so staff can quickly recognize it. Assign personnel to check emergency supplies regularly. Replace and discard expired medication and equipment. Run anaphylaxis drills regularly, and most important of all: Keep calm and give epinephrine.

34.2 An Ounce of Prevention

While it's impossible to avoid all potential situations that could lead to anaphylaxis (other than not practicing allergy), there are certain measures that can be taken to help reduce or minimize the risk of a serious reaction occurring.

- Select appropriate candidates for skin testing and immunotherapy. See
  ► Table 34.1 for a list of patients who may be at increased risk of adverse reactions.
- To help minimize human error have systems in place; double-check vial prescriptions and mixing notes. Double confirm patients' identities and read back information on each vial to confirm it is the right vial for the right patient; double-check dosage prior to shot administration.
- Have standard operating procedure (SOP) for testing, mixing, and shot administration. Review them with staff periodically, ensure they are following it, and that new staff are trained properly on it.

Table 34.1 Patients at increased risk for serious allergic reactions

- Patients who've had a prior serious reaction or episode of anaphylaxis

- Uncontrolled or poorly controlled asthmatics

- Patients on certain medications that increase risk or complicate treatment:

  ○ Beta blockers

  ○ Angiotensin converting enzyme inhibitors

  ○ Angiotensin blockers

  ○ Tricyclic antidepressants (select)

- Very young children

- Testing/treating very sensitive patients when their allergen is "in season"

34.3 Prepare for the Worst

- Establish an anaphylaxis protocol in the clinic. Post it in all patient treatment rooms or allergy patient care areas. See ▶ Fig. 34.1 for an example of a protocol.

If your anaphylaxis protocol does not clearly list medications and dosages, post a list of emergency medications with dosages as well. If you treat kids, post pediatric doses or mg/kg.

- Keep an allergy emergency cart or anaphylaxis kit/cart (▶ Fig. 34.2a, b; ▶ Fig. 34.3).
- Perform anaphylaxis drills at periodic intervals.
- Assign personnel to check emergency supplies and replace/discard outdated equipment/medications.
- Have a predetermined method of communication (calling for help, walkie talkies, intercom) for emergencies and designate in advance the roles staff play (who calls 911, etc.)

Anaphylaxis Protocol: ADULTS AND CHILDREN

When multiple options are listed for a step, the first medication, dose, route is preferred

STEPS:

1. **Remove** the inciting allergen, if possible.

2. **Assess** airway, breathing, circulation, and orientation; if needed, support the airway using the

   least invasive but effective method (eg, bag-valve-mask)

3. Start CPR/chest compressions (100/min) if cardiovascular arrest occurs at any time

4. **Inject epinephrine and may repeat Q5-15** minutes as indicated:

   Use auto-injector in lateral thigh — **0.3mg** injector for Adults and Children greater than 65 lbs

   0.15mg injector for Children 65 lbs or less

   Alternative, 1:1,000 epinephrine from ampule. Dose is 0.3 – 0.5 mg (0.01 mg /kg for children) intramuscularly in lateral thigh

   If inadequate response to IM injection[s], give epinephrine by continuous infusion by micro-drip Or infusion pump; add 1 mg (1 ml of 1:1,000) of epinephrine to 1 L of 0.9 NL saline;

   Start infusion at 2 microg/min (2 mL/min = 120 mL/h) and increase up to 10 microg/min (10 mL/min = 600 mL/h); titrate dose with continuous monitoring

5. **GET HELP!** Summon appropriate assistance in office and call 911

6. Place adults and adolescents in recumbent **position;** place young children in position of comfort;

   Place pregnant patient on left side

7. **Oxygen:**

   If SpO2 95-100%, give via nasal cannula at **2-4** lpm

   If SpO2 90-95%, give via simple face mask at **8-10** L/min

   If SpO2 less than 90%, give via non-rebreather face mask at **15** lpm

8. **Establish IV** for fluid replacement; keep open with 0.9 NL saline, push fluids at **wide open rate** for blood pressure less than 100/60 or up to **30 mL/kg** in first hour for children.

   Caution with patients with a known history of volume overload, such as CHF or renal disease

ADDITIONAL MEASURES

8. **H1 Antihistamine**—give **25-50** mg of diphenhydramine IM for adults and **1mg/kg** (maximum 50 mg) for children;

   Alternative, use **10** mg of cetirizine [Zyrtec] orally

9. If Wheezing or trouble breathing, give **Albuterol 2 puffs** via MDI; repeat prn Q15 minutes

   Alternative: 2.5-5 mg of nebulized albuterol in 3 mL of saline; repeat PRN Q15 min

Fig. 34.1 An example of an office anaphylaxis protocol.

10. FOR PATIENTS ON B-BLOCKERS:

If not responding to epinephrine, give **1-5 mg of Glucagon** intravenously slowly over 5 min

> CAUTION: rapid administration of glucagon can induce vomiting

12. <u>If reaction is following a subcutaneous injection,</u> place tourniquet above injection site. Can also inject 1-2 mL of 1% lidocaine with epinephrine 1:100,000 at the site of injection

13. Steroids:

> Methylprednisolone: 1-2 mg/kg up to 125 mg per dose, IM, IV [diluted in 10 ml of NS], or orally

> Decadron: 10-20 mg IM/IV adults, 4-10 mg IM/IV children

Fig. 34.1 (*Continued*)

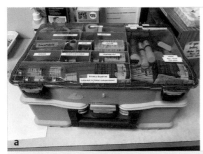 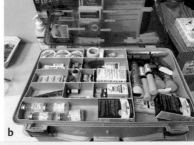

Fig. 34.2 (a) An anaphylaxis kit. It should be kept unlocked, in a place that is easily accessible by staff, and restocked regularly. **(b)** Medications inside an anaphylaxis kit. Be sure to discard and replace expired medication.

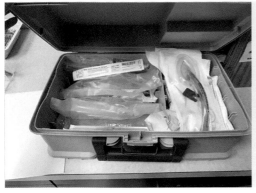

Fig. 34.3 Airway and other supplies that may be present in an anaphylaxis kit.

34.4 When Anaphylaxis Strikes

The first step is to identify potential or suspected anaphylaxis. If you think it might be anaphylaxis, treat it like it is anaphylaxis until it proves to be otherwise. ▶ Table 34.2 lists some signs and symptoms of anaphylaxis.

Suspect anaphylaxis if:

- The patient has been exposed to an allergen and develops two or more symptoms from ▶ Table 34.2.
- The patient develops skin/mucosal symptoms with either respiratory symptoms or hypotension.
- After allergen exposure, hypotension develops.

If anaphylaxis is suspected, begin treatment following your protocol. Important steps to take are:

1. Remove any inciting allergen (if feasible), assess patient, start cardiopulmonary resuscitation (CPR) if indicated.
2. Inject epinephrine. See ▶ Table 34.3 for dosages; may repeat every 5 to 15 minutes as indicated.
3. Call 911 (or local emergency number). Get help! Summon additional nursing/office assistance.
4. Place patient in supine position or comfortable position if airway issues. Pregnant patients are positioned on their left side.
5. Give oxygen. See ▶ Table 34.3.
6. If hypotensive, place intravenous (IV) line and give fluids.
7. For wheezing/dyspnea not improved by epinephrine, give albuterol. See ▶ Table 34.3.

Table 34.2 Signs and symptoms of anaphylaxis

Skin	Respiratory
• Hives, angioedema	• Wheezing, coughing, throat clearing
• Itching without hives/rash	• Difficulty breathing, runny nose
• Flushing	• Upper aerodigestive tract angioedema
Blood pressure changes	**Abdominal/gastrointestinal**
• Hypotension, syncope	• Nausea, vomiting, diarrhea
• Dizziness, sweating	• Abdominal pain
Other symptoms	
"Feeling of doom," headache, incontinence, seizure, confusion, metallic taste in mouth	

Table 34.3 Doses of medications that can be given as part of an anaphylaxis protocol

Epinephrine

- Administer in lateral thigh

- Auto-injector: 0.3-mg injector for patients > 65 lbs; 0.15-mg injector for patients 65–33 lbs; 0.1-mg injector (if available) for 33–16.5 lbs

- 1:1,000 epinephrine ampule: 0.3–0.5 mg (0.01 mg/kg for children) IM

- Continuous infusion by micro-drip or infusion pump: Add 1 mg (1 mL of 1:1,000) of epinephrine to 1 L of 0.9 NL saline; start infusion at 2 µg/min (2 mL/min = 120 mL/h) and increase up to 10 µg/min (10 mL/min = 600 mL/h); titrate dose with continuous monitoring

Oxygen

- If SpO_2 95–100%, give via nasal cannula at 2–4 L/min

- If SpO_2 90–95%, give via simple face mask at 8–10 L/min

- If SpO_2 < 90%, give via non-rebreather face mask at 15 L/min

IV fluid replacement

- 0.9 NS to run in, push fluids at wide open rate for blood pressure < 100/60 or up to 30 mL/kg in first hour for children[a]

H1 Antihistamine

- Diphenhydramine: Give 25–50 mg IM for adults and 1 mg/kg (max 50 mg) for children.
- Alternatively, use 10 mg of cetirizine/loratadine orally

Beta-2 Agonist

- Albuterol: 2–4 puffs via MDI; repeat PRN every 15 min
- Alternative: 2.5–5 mg of nebulized albuterol in 3 mL of saline; repeat PRN every 15 min

Steroids

- Methylprednisolone: 1–2 mg/kg up to 125 mg per dose, IM, IV (diluted in 10 mL of NS), or orally
- Decadron: 10–20 mg IM/IV for adults, 4–10 mg IM/IV for children

Glucagon

- 1–5 mg IV slowly over 5 min[b]

Abbreviations: IM, intramuscularly; IV, intravenously; MDI, metered-dose inhaler; NS, normal saline; PRN, as needed; SpO_2, blood oxygen saturation.
[a]Be cautious with patients with a known history of volume overload, such as congestive heart failure (CHF) or renal disease.
[b]Caution: Rapid administration of glucagon can induce vomiting.

Additional treatment considerations:
- H1 antihistamines (i.e., diphenhydramine). See ▶ Table 34.3 for dosing.
- Corticosteroids (i.e., methylprednisolone). See ▶ Table 34.3 for dosing.
- For patients on beta blockers unresponsive to epinephrine, give glucagon. See ▶ Table 34.3.

> Caution with glucagon administration. Rapid administration can induce vomiting.

34.5 A Word About Epinephrine

Anaphylaxis does occur in a spectrum, from mild to extremely severe. There are grading scales to rate the severity of anaphylaxis and they do include mild grades of anaphylaxis. Epinephrine can and should be used to treat all forms of anaphylaxis and early administration of epinephrine saves lives. Epinephrine is the only thing that has been shown to improve survival in episodes of anaphylaxis, and it may need to be administered more than once. Despite the facts that there are no absolute contraindications to epinephrine administration and that early use of epinephrine saves lives, this medication has acquired the stigma that it is a "serious" medication and anaphylaxis has to be "severe enough" to give it. Unfortunately, there is no way to predict which episodes of mild anaphylaxis will progress and which won't. If you suspect you have a patient in anaphylaxis and think about giving epinephrine, don't wait—give epinephrine.

34.6 Hope for the Best

After any adverse allergic event or anaphylaxis (even mild cases), it's helpful to hold a "debrief." This can be done immediately after an event or in a meeting format where all events that occur in a day/week/month are reviewed. Discuss the event or events with the staff—what went well, what could be improved, any obstacles that were encountered, and anything else that could have prevented or improved the situation. These debriefs can be helpful in fine-tuning, updating, or changing procedures currently in practice, so that future adverse events can be prevented.

Clinical Pearls   M!

- Be prepared with an anaphylaxis protocol—post it, practice it, plan for it
- Be sure to have emergency supplies and unexpired medication.
- Know the possible symptoms of anaphylaxis—if you think it might be anaphylaxis, treat it like anaphylaxis until proven otherwise.
- Epinephrine, epinephrine, epinephrine. It saves lives. Give it early for any confirmed or suspected case of anaphylaxis. If you think about giving epinephrine, give epinephrine.
- Hold a debrief—learn what went well, look at ways to improve what didn't.

Bibliography

[1] Campbell RL, Li JTC, Nicklas RA, Sadosty AT, Members of the Joint Task Force, Practice Parameter Workgroup. Emergency department diagnosis and treatment of anaphylaxis: a practice parameter. Ann Allergy Asthma Immunol. 2014; 113(6):599–608

[2] Lieberman P, Nicklas RA, Randolph C, et al. Anaphylaxis–a practice parameter update 2015. Ann Allergy Asthma Immunol. 2015; 115(5):341–384

35 Other Urgencies and Emergencies

Christine B. Franzese

35.1 A Horse with Stripes

One of the author's partners is fond of saying, "Sometimes it's not a zebra, sometimes it's just a horse with stripes." While anaphylaxis is something every allergy practice must be prepared to treat, fortunately it's fairly uncommon. There are other adverse events that can happen with higher frequency that the clinician also needs to be prepared to recognize and treat. Some of these reactions are similar to or can mimic anaphylaxis. Some of them can be part of an anaphylactic reaction. Establishing protocols and educating not only yourself, but your allergy and office staff, on early recognition and the steps to take to manage/treat these other reactions will help your office be prepared to handle whatever manner of equine should present itself that day.

35.2 Local Reactions

Local reactions come in two types: Immediate or delayed.
- **Immediate:** Occur within an hour of subcutaneous immunotherapy (SCIT) injection; frequently seen.
- **Delayed:** Occur 8 to 24 hours after SCIT injection or skin testing; frequently seen.

Symptoms include swelling of variable size, redness, itching at the site of the injection/testing area.

Both types can be treated with oral antihistamines, ice, and topical corticosteroid ointments. Premedication with an oral antihistamine prior to injection can help.

> I have my patients premedicate with the oral antihistamine of their choice either the evening prior or morning of their SCIT injection. It is also helpful to educate patients on what local reactions are and their signs/symptoms.

Large local reactions result in more than 30 mm in diameter (larger than half-dollar coin) and patients should be instructed to report their occurrence. Although repeated large local reactions show no tendency to progress to systemic reactions, some providers will adjust the dose of SCIT for these large reactions.

35.3 Vasovagal Reaction

These reactions can mimic systemic allergic reactions and frequently seen during testing and injections.

Symptoms include low/normal blood pressure, sweating, pallor, weakness, nausea, and vomiting.

This reaction may result in a brief loss of consciousness, and even tonic-clonic movements but there should be no loss of bowel or bladder control. Patients describe themselves as "feeling woozy/faint/dizzy," but do not have an impending sense of doom. They may even state their feelings such as they are going to pass out. Pulse is generally slow and blood pressure is normal when supine or reclined. Distinguished from anaphylaxis by no skin manifestations (hives, swelling, itching, and flushing).

This reaction is treated with monitoring, symptomatic support (cold washcloth/compress, place in supine position), reassurance, and an ammonia ampoule, if needed.

35.4 Asthma Exacerbation

This can be part of an anaphylactic reaction. More common in poorly compliant, poorly controlled, or "in season" asthmatics.

Symptoms include wheezing, coughing, and chest tightness.

While an isolated asthma exacerbation can occur after injection, be certain with careful monitoring and frequent symptom assessment that wheezing or chest tightness is not progressing or accompanied by other symptoms as described in Chapter 34.

Treatment is with albuterol, either by metered-dose inhaler and/or nebulizer.

Patients should be instructed to report any asthma exacerbations or albuterol use prior to testing or injection. After an acute exacerbation, the provider should evaluate the patient's current medication compliance and determine if medication adjustment is indicated. Consideration should be given to whether the patient's SCIT dosage needs to be adjusted as well.

> Spirometry prior to testing and having the patient perform a peak-flow or fraction of exhaled nitrous (FeNO) test prior to injection can also be helpful.

35.5 Isolated Urticaria

This can be part of an anaphylactic reaction; uncommon to rare; more likely to happen in patients with chronic or physical urticarias on SCIT.

Symptoms include hives, variable in size, location, and number.

While an isolated urticarial outbreak can occur after injection, be certain with careful monitoring and frequent symptom assessment that hives are not progressing or accompanied by other symptoms describe in Chapter 35.

Treatment is with oral or intramuscular antihistamines. Consideration can be given to oral or injected corticosteroids.

Patients with a history of chronic/physical urticarias should be instructed to report any hives prior to testing or injection. After an acute outbreak of hives, the provider should evaluate the patient's current medication compliance and if medication adjustment is indicated. Consideration should be given to whether the patient's SCIT dosage needs to be adjusted as well.

35.6 Chest Pain/Hypoglycemia/Other Symptoms Not Related to Anaphylaxis

Uncommon to rare; may occur completely unrelated to SCIT or testing.

Symptoms are variable, depending on disorder/disease process.

Treatment is variable but generally it is better to call 911 and provide symptomatic support until help arrives.

Clinical Pearls M!

- Educate patients on local reactions, premedicate if needed/desired.
- Patients should report local reactions, asthma exacerbations, hives, pregnancy, any other illness prior to getting injections or testing.
- Acute exacerbations of asthma or hives with injections require reassessment of the patient's medication regimen.
- Vasovagal reactions are very common; be sure to distinguish these from anaphylaxis.

Bibliography

[1] Cox L, Nelson H, Lockey R, et al. Allergen immunotherapy: a practice parameter third update. J Allergy Clin Immunol. 2011; 127(1) Suppl:S1–S55

[2] Lieberman P, Nicklas RA, Randolph C, et al. Anaphylaxis–a practice parameter update 2015. Ann Allergy Asthma Immunol. 2015; 115(5):341–384

Part 6

Associated Atopic Disorders

36 Penicillin Allergy

Christine B. Franzese

36.1 Fear and Labelling

It might seem unusual to think of penicillin (PCN) allergy as terrifying but when treating a patient with PCN allergy who has an infection, a lot of fear is generated. Some on the part of the practitioner (What can I use to treat the patient with? Are cephalosporins safe? What happens if the patient has a serious reaction?), and some on the part of the patient (My mother had a serious reaction to penicillin, she told everyone in the family not to take it!). It's also an extremely difficult label to get off of a patient's medical chart and will follow the patient around the health care system, even if incorrect. The author has come across patients who have got the label added to their chart even when they do not have any adverse reaction to penicillin, and they are afraid to remove it. Adding PCN allergy testing to a practice can help not only the patient, but also colleagues, and help reduce the overall cost of health care.

36.2 Serious Stuff

PCN allergy is classified as Type B (unpredictable) adverse drug reaction. It can manifest as any of the Gell and Coombs hypersensitivity reactions. Type I (IgE-mediated, immediate hypersensitivity) and Type IV (cell-mediated, delayed) reactions are the most common.

- Type I IgE-mediated hypersensitivity typically occurs soon after exposure and includes hives, swelling, itching, and angioedema.
- Type IV IgE-mediated hypersensitivity typically occurs toward the end of exposure and includes drug rashes, toxic epidermal necrolysis (TEN), and Steven-Johnsons syndrome.

Of the general population only 10% report an allergy to PCN and 90% are found to tolerate it.

> PCN allergy is not fixed. Roughly 50–60% of patients with IgE-mediated PCN allergy will lose it after 5 years; 90% or more will lose it after 10 years.

36.3 History

How can a practitioner identify candidates for PCN allergy testing? Unfortunately, a practitioner has to talk to people and ask them questions. Here are some questions that are helpful to ask:

- What type of PCN was given? What was the route of administration?
- What was the reason it was given?
- What was the reaction?
- When in the course of the medication did the reaction happen? How long ago was it?
- How was the reaction treated?
- Have you had PCN since then? Have you had a cephalosporin since then?
  - Answers that are consistent with an IgE-mediated PCN allergy (hives, happened soon after starting PCN) are candidates for testing.
  - Many patients will not know what the reaction was ("I was an infant, my mother told me I was allergic")] or will report he/she is allergic to PCN when never having taken it due to a family member having a PCN allergy. These patients are also potential candidates for testing.

36.4 Diagnosis and Testing

Specific IgE testing is not recommended.

If IgE tests are negative, cannot tell patient he/she does not have PCN allergy. Seriously, what good is that?

- Prick testing, followed by intradermal testing is recommended (followed by optional oral challenge).

> If patient has an adverse reaction to PCN testing, it is generally no worse than the initial reaction. If the initial reaction was hives, then any adverse reaction during testing is generally no worse than hives.

36.5 Shocking Information—How to Actually Do This!

- **Step 1:** Prick testing consists of placing four prick tests. A single positive control (histamine), a single negative control (saline), a single penicillin G (at 1:10,000 u/mL), and a single benzylpenicilloyl polylysine (PrePen) are applied using single prick devices (▶ Fig. 36.1).

○ Results are read at 15 to 20 minutes

○ If controls are valid, a positive test at either the PCN G or PrePen site indicates PCN allergy and testing stops. Patient is informed to avoid PCN.

○ If controls are valid, negative tests at both the PCN G and PrePen sites indicate patient can proceed to Step 2.

Note: PrePen is the only commercially available penicilloyl extract in the United States at present.

• **Step 2:** Intradermal testing consists of placing five intradermal tests, each 3 mm in size. A single negative control (saline), two penicillin G (at 1:10,000 u/mL), and two PrePen intradermal tests are placed using the intradermal technique described in Chapter 16.

A 3-mm otoscope makes a perfect 3-mm circle—useful for busy allergy nurses (▶ Fig. 36.2).

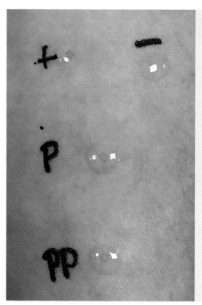

Fig. 36.1 Step 1—skin prick testing (SPT) for penicillin (PCN) allergy.

○ Results are read at 10 to 15 minutes.
○ A positive test is growth of wheal 2 to 3 mm greater than the negative control.

It is helpful to draw a circle outlining the initial wheal so that any growth is easier to see (▶ Fig. 36.3).

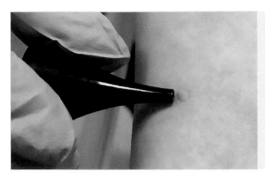

Fig. 36.2 A 3-mm otoscope sheath imprint on skin.

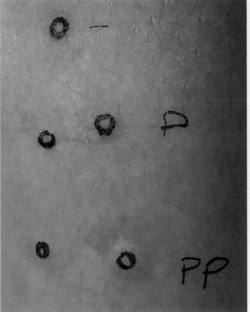

Fig. 36.3 Step 2—intradermal testing for penicillin (PCN) allergy. Initial wheals are outlined with marker for clarity. Note positive test results at PrePen sites.

- ○ If all four testing sites are negative, patient can proceed to an oral challenge.
- ○ If both PCN G or PrePen sites are positive (as shown in ▶ Fig. 36.3), then testing is stopped and patient is informed to avoid PCN.
- ○ If one PCN G and/or PrePen site is positive and the other is negative, then a single additional intradermal injection is placed of PCN G (if it was positive) and/or PrePen (if it was positive). The additional test is read at 10 to 15 minutes and the results of two out of three tests determine the result. If there are two negative tests, the patient proceeds to an oral challenge. If there are two positives, then testing stops and patient is told to avoid PCN.
- **Step 3:** Oral challenge—if prick and intradermal tests are negative, an oral challenge can be performed at this point.
  - ○ It is considered optional, but up to 20% of PCN allergy patients may have negative skin tests.
  - ○ Oral challenge procedure varies. One protocol is to give the patient a single 250-mg dose of PCN VK and have them wait for 60 minutes. If no reaction, patient is then given a single 250-mg dose of amoxicillin and asked to wait another for 60 minutes. Another protocol is to give a 25-mg dose (1/10th of initial dose—elixir is helpful here) and to wait for 30 to 60 minutes. If no reaction, then proceed with 250 mg of PCN, followed by 250 mg of amoxicillin if no reaction after 60 minutes with the 250-mg dose of PCN.

A patient can be only allergic to amoxicillin, and can take other PCNs safely. If there is a reaction, the patient is told to avoid amoxicillin. If no reaction, patient is cleared to take all PCNs.

Clinical Pearls   M!

- If tests are negative, patient should be given copy of testing results.
- Resensitization rates to PCN are very low, roughly 0–3%. Resensitization is most common after high-dose PCN treatment and consideration to retesting may be given.
- If tests are positive, patient should avoid PCN; however, consideration to retesting can be given in 5 years or more.

Bibliography

[1] Fox SJ, Park MA. Penicillin skin testing is a safe and effective tool for evaluating penicillin allergy in the pediatric population. J Allergy Clin Immunol Pract. 2014; 2(4):439–444

[2] Joint Task Force on Practice Parameters, American Academy of Allergy, Asthma and Immunology, American College of Allergy, Asthma and Immunology, Joint Council of Allergy, Asthma and Immunology. Drug allergy: an updated practice parameter. Ann Allergy Asthma Immunol. 2010; 105(4):259–273

[3] Penicillin Skin Testing. Available at https://www.uptodate.com/contents/penicillin-skin-testing. Accessed at May 22, 2019

37 Asthma

Christine B. Franzese

37.1 More Than Just Wheezing

Asthma is one of the most common associated comorbid conditions seen in an allergy practice. The practitioner should have a basic understanding of asthma. The author's understanding of asthma has evolved from just a disorder of bronchoconstriction to realizing that lower airway inflammation, tissue remodeling, and airway hyperresponsiveness play a role as well. In addition, different phenotypes/endotypes of asthma, how to recognize or evaluate asthmatic patients for different phenotypes/endotypes, and what treatment each type of asthma responds best to is now being recognized and explored. It would be impossible to adequately cover asthma diagnosis, testing, and treatment in one chapter. However, even if a practitioner decides not to participate in asthma management in allergy practice, he/she should assess both their level of severity and current level of control when testing or treating asthmatic patients with immunotherapy. This chapter will focus on assessing a patient's asthma severity and control.

37.2 How Bad It Can Get

Asthma severity is statement about the baseline quality of the patient's asthma. It is easiest to assess in a patient newly diagnosed with asthma who's not on long-term controller medication, but even if that patient is currently on controller medications, you can get an idea of the patient's baseline severity level by the current medications being used to keep them in control. The National Heart, Lung, and Blood Institute (NHLBI) 2007 guidelines for the diagnosis and treatment of asthma includes recommendations on how to assess a patient's level of asthma severity. ▶ Fig. 37.1 from the NHLBI is a quick reference guide on assessing asthma severity by asking the patient about symptom frequency, nighttime awakening, use of short-acting controller medications such as albuterol, interference with normal activity, and any spirometry or pulmonary function testing results, if available.

> Asthmatic patients are notorious about under-reporting or under-recognizing the impact their symptoms are having on their daily lives and will frequently adjust their daily activities to fit within their current level of symptoms, rather than recognizing the impact it's having upon them. Be sure to keep this in mind when questioning asthmatic patients about any limitations in daily activities.

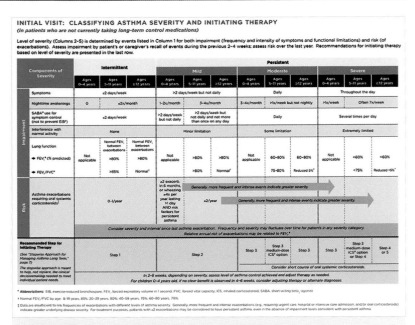

INITIAL VISIT: CLASSIFYING ASTHMA SEVERITY AND INITIATING THERAPY
(in patients who are not currently taking long-term control medications)

Level of severity (Columns 2-5) is determined by events listed in Column 1 for both impairment (frequency and intensity of symptoms and functional limitations) and risk (of exacerbations). Assess impairment by patient's or caregiver's recall of events during the previous 2-4 weeks; assess risk over the last year. Recommendations for initiating therapy based on level of severity are presented in the last row.

Fig. 37.1 Guidelines for assessing asthma severity and initiating therapy.
Source: National Heart, Lung and Blood Institute.

Asthma is generally categorized as intermittent or persistent, and within the persistent category further subdivided into mild, moderate, or severe. Once categorized, the NHLBI guidelines provide recommendations for asthma therapy in a step-wise approach seen in ▶ Fig. 37.2.

37.3 Control

Asthma is a dynamic disease and periodically assessing a patient's control is a necessary part of any allergy practice, if a practitioner is treating any patients with comorbid asthma. Asthma control is generally categorized by being either well-controlled, not well-controlled, or very poorly controlled. The assessment and categorization of a patient's level of control is based on patient responses to questions that are similar to those used to assess severity. That is, questions about frequency of symptoms, nighttime awakenings, responses to quality-of-life questionnaires related to asthma, use of short-acting controller medications such as albuterol, interference with normal activity, and any spirometry or pulmonary function testing results, if available. Depending on the patient's responses and any test results available, you can use ▶ Fig. 37.3 to help

STEPWISE APPROACH FOR MANAGING ASTHMA LONG TERM

The stepwise approach tailors the selection of medication to the level of asthma severity (see page 5) or asthma control (see page 6). The stepwise approach is meant to help, not replace, the clinical decisionmaking needed to meet individual patient needs.

ASSESS CONTROL:

STEP UP IF NEEDED (first, check medication adherence, inhaler technique, environmental control, and comorbidities)

STEP DOWN IF POSSIBLE (and asthma is well controlled for at least 3 months)

		STEP 1	STEP 2	STEP 3	STEP 4	STEP 5	STEP 6
		At each step: Patient education, environmental control, and management of comorbidities					
0–4 years of age		Intermittent Asthma	Persistent Asthma: Daily Medication Consult with asthma specialist if step 3 care or higher is required. Consider consultation at step 2.				
	Preferred Treatment[†]	SABA* as needed	low-dose ICS*	medium-dose ICS*	medium-dose ICS* + either LABA* or montelukast	high-dose ICS* + either LABA* or montelukast	high-dose ICS* + either LABA* or montelukast + oral corticosteroids
	Alternative Treatment[†‡]		cromolyn or montelukast				
		If clear benefit is not observed in 4–6 weeks, and medication technique and adherence are satisfactory, consider adjusting therapy or alternate diagnoses.					
	Quick-Relief Medication	• SABA* as needed for symptoms; intensity of treatment depends on severity of symptoms. • With viral respiratory symptoms: SABA every 4-6 hours up to 24 hours (longer with physician consult). Consider short course of oral systemic corticosteroids if asthma exacerbation is severe or patient has history of severe exacerbations. • Caution: Frequent use of SABA may indicate the need to step up treatment.					
5–11 years of age		Intermittent Asthma	Persistent Asthma: Daily Medication Consult with asthma specialist if step 4 care or higher is required. Consider consultation at step 3.				
	Preferred Treatment[†]	SABA* as needed	low-dose ICS*	low-dose ICS* + either LABA,* LTRA,* or theophylline[§] OR medium-dose ICS	medium-dose ICS* + LABA*	high-dose ICS* + LABA*	high-dose ICS* + LABA* + oral corticosteroids
	Alternative Treatment[†‡]		cromolyn, LTRA,* or theophylline[§]		medium-dose ICS* + either LTRA* or theophylline[§]	high-dose ICS* + either LTRA* or theophylline[§]	high-dose ICS* + either LTRA* or theophylline[§] + oral corticosteroids
		Consider subcutaneous allergen immunotherapy for patients who have persistent, allergic asthma.**					
	Quick-Relief Medication	• SABA* as needed for symptoms. The intensity of treatment depends on severity of symptoms: up to 3 treatments every 20 minutes as needed. Short course of oral systemic corticosteroids may be needed. • Caution: Increasing use of SABA or use >2 days/week for symptom relief (not to prevent EIB*) generally indicates inadequate control and the need to step up treatment.					
≥12 years of age		Intermittent Asthma	Persistent Asthma: Daily Medication Consult with asthma specialist if step 4 care or higher is required. Consider consultation at step 3.				
	Preferred Treatment[†]	SABA* as needed	low-dose ICS*	low-dose ICS* + LABA* OR medium-dose ICS*	medium-dose ICS* + LABA*	high-dose ICS* + LABA* AND consider omalizumab for patients who have allergies**	high-dose ICS* + LABA* + oral corticosteroid[§§] AND consider omalizumab for patients who have allergies**
	Alternative Treatment[†‡]		cromolyn, LTRA,* or theophylline[§]	low-dose ICS* + either LTRA,* theophylline,[§] or zileuton[‡‡]	medium-dose ICS* + either LTRA,* theophylline,[§] or zileuton[‡‡]		
		Consider subcutaneous allergen immunotherapy for patients who have persistent, allergic asthma.**					
	Quick-Relief Medication	• SABA* as needed for symptoms. The intensity of treatment depends on severity of symptoms: up to 3 treatments every 20 minutes as needed. Short course of oral systemic corticosteroids may be needed. • Caution: Use of SABA >2 days/week for symptom relief (not to prevent EIB*) generally indicates inadequate control and the need to step up treatment.					

* **Abbreviations:** EIB, exercise-induced bronchospasm; ICS, inhaled corticosteroid; LABA, inhaled long-acting beta₂-agonist; LTRA, leukotriene receptor antagonist; SABA, inhaled short-acting beta₂-agonist

[†] Treatment options are listed in alphabetical order, if more than one.

[‡] If alternative treatment is used and response is inadequate, discontinue and use preferred treatment before stepping up.

[§] Theophylline is a less desirable alternative because of the need to monitor serum concentration levels.

** Based on evidence for dust mites, animal dander, and pollen; evidence is weak or lacking for molds and cockroaches. Evidence is strongest for immunotherapy with single allergens. The role of allergy in asthma is greater in children than in adults.

** Clinicians who administer immunotherapy or omalizumab should be prepared to treat anaphylaxis that may occur.

[‡‡] Zileuton is less desirable because of limited studies as adjunctive therapy and the need to monitor liver function.

[§§] Before oral corticosteroids are introduced, a trial of high-dose ICS + LABA + either LTRA, theophylline, or zileuton, may be considered, although this approach has not been studied in clinical trials.

Fig. 37.2 Stepwise guidelines for managing asthma.
Source: National Heart, Lung and Blood Institute.

FOLLOW-UP VISITS: ASSESSING ASTHMA CONTROL AND ADJUSTING THERAPY

Level of control (Columns 2-4) is based on the most severe component of impairment (symptoms and functional limitations) or risk (exacerbations). Assess impairment by patient's or caregiver's recall of events listed in Column 1 during the previous 2-4 weeks and by spirometry and/or peak flow measures. Symptom assessment for longer periods should reflect a global assessment, such as inquiring whether the patient's asthma is better or worse since the last visit. Assess risk by recall of exacerbations during the previous year and since the last visit. Recommendations for adjusting therapy based on level of control are presented in the last row.

	Components of Control	Well Controlled			Not Well Controlled			Very Poorly Controlled		
		Ages 0-4 years	Ages 5-11 years	Ages ≥12 years	Ages 0-4 years	Ages 5-11 years	Ages ≥12 years	Ages 0-4 years	Ages 5-11 years	Ages ≥12 years
Impairment	Symptoms	≤2 days/week	≤2 days/week but not more than once on each day	≤2 days/week	>2 days/week	>2 days/week or multiple times on ≤2 days/week	>2 days/week	Throughout the day		
	Nighttime awakenings	≤1x/month		≤2x/month	>1x/month	≥2x/month	1-3x/week	>1x/week	≥2x/week	≥4x/week
	Interference with normal activity	None			Some limitation			Extremely limited		
	SABA* use for symptom control (not to prevent EIB*)	≤2 days/week			>2 days/week			Several times per day		
	Lung function • FEV_1* (% predicted) or peak flow (% personal best)	Not applicable	>80%	>80%	Not applicable	60-80%	60-80%	Not applicable	<60%	<60%
	• FEV_1/FVC*		>80%	Not applicable		75-80%	Not applicable		<75%	Not applicable
	Validated questionnaires† • ATAQ* • ACQ* • ACT*	Not applicable	Not applicable	0 ≤0.75‡ ≥20	Not applicable	Not applicable	1-2 ≥1.5 16-19	Not applicable	Not applicable	3-4 Not applicable ≤15
Risk	Asthma exacerbations requiring oral systemic corticosteroids§	0-1/year			2-3/year	≥2/year		>3/year	≥2/year	
		Consider severity and interval since last asthma exacerbation.								
	Reduction in lung growth/Progressive loss of lung function	Not applicable	Evaluation requires long-term follow-up care.		Not applicable	Evaluation requires long-term follow-up care.		Not applicable	Evaluation requires long-term follow-up care.	
	Treatment-related adverse effects	*Medication side effects can vary in intensity from none to very troublesome and worrisome. The level of intensity does not correlate to specific levels of control but should be considered in the overall assessment of risk.*								
Recommended Action for Treatment *(See "Stepwise Approach for Managing Asthma Long Term," page 7)* *The stepwise approach is meant to help, not replace, the clinical decisionmaking needed to meet individual patient needs.*		*Maintain current step.* *Regular follow-up every 1-6 months.* *Consider step down if well controlled for at least 3 months.*			Step up 1 step	Step up at least 1 step	Step up 1 step	*Consider short course of oral systemic corticosteroids.* *Step up 1-2 steps.* *Reevaluate in 2 weeks to achieve control.*		
					Reevaluate in 2-6 weeks to achieve control. *For children 0-4 years, if no clear benefit observed in 4-6 weeks, consider adjusting therapy or alternative diagnoses.*					
					Before step up in treatment: *Review adherence to medication, inhaler technique, and environmental control. If alternative treatment was used, discontinue and use preferred treatment for that step. For side effects, consider alternative treatment options.*					

* **Abbreviations:** ACQ, Asthma Control Questionnaire©; ACT, Asthma Control Test™; ATAQ, Asthma Therapy Assessment Questionnaire©; EIB, exercise-induced bronchospasm; FVC, forced vital capacity; FEV_1, forced expiratory volume in 1 second; SABA, short-acting $beta_2$-agonist

† Minimal important difference: 1.0 for the ATAQ; 0.5 for the ACQ; not determined for the ACT.

‡ ACQ values of 0.76-1.4 are indeterminate regarding well-controlled asthma.

§ Data are insufficient to link frequencies of exacerbations with different levels of asthma control. Generally, more frequent and intense exacerbations (e.g., requiring urgent care, hospital or intensive care admission, and/or oral corticosteroids) indicate poorer asthma control.

Fig. 37.3 Guidelines for assessing asthma control and adjusting therapy. Source: National Heart, Lung and Blood Institute.

determine the patient's level of current asthma control and what, if any, changes in treatment should be made if the patient's asthma is being treated or whether the patient needs to be referred back to his/her asthma care provider, sooner rather than later. Any "step up" references in ▶ Fig. 37.3 are referring back to the step-wise asthma treatment guidelines shown in ▶ Fig. 37.2.

Remember—asthmatics are notorious for downplaying or minimizing exacerbations and forgetting the impact their symptoms play in their daily lives. Be sure to keep this in mind when assessing current asthma control and be sure to ask direct questions about specific activities the patient does or use an asthma assessment questionnaire.

37.4 The Undiagnosed

Often patients with undiagnosed asthma come to clinic for immunotherapy. Be suspicious of it and look for it. Some asthmatic patients may not always have had adequate access to care, or have been inadvertently diagnosed with other disorders, or may just be in denial. Making the diagnosis (or confirming your suspected diagnoses) is extremely important, not only if a practitioner or the patient is thinking of allergy skin testing or immunotherapy, but also for the patient's overall health. As a patient, proper asthma treatment can improve the one's quality of life and make any immunotherapy received less fraught with exacerbations and adverse reactions. As an allergy practitioner, ensuring the patient has proper asthma treatment can help reduce any additional risks of severe adverse reactions, exacerbations, or anaphylaxis and help properly prepare the patient and office staff if the worst should occur.

While assessing a new patient and elicit a history of wheezing, coughing, chest tightness, or recurrent breathing problems, or the patient states these symptoms occur or worsen with exercise, changes in temperature, weather, or exposure to allergens, viruses, or other factors, this should trigger the "potential asthma diagnosis" alarm bell in practitioner's mind. Obtain spirometry in office or refer the patient for pulmonary function testing. Treat these potential alarm bells similar to how treat anaphylaxis should be treated or using epinephrine: if you think the patient has anaphylaxis, treat the patient like he/she does; if you think about using epinephrine, use epinephrine. For these patients, if you think there's a possibility they might have asthma, send them for testing and treat them like they do have asthma.

37.5 The Future Understanding of Asthma

As mentioned at the beginning of the chapter, physicians have started to appreciate that asthma comes in a variety of different flavors, or phenotypes, and that it is not just a single disease with a single pathophysiologic mechanism, but a host of different endotypes with different underlying pathologies and differing responses to medical therapies. The practitioners are also beginning to understand the influence a patient's genotype has on the expression on his/her type of asthma and what response (or lack thereof) the patient may have to controller medications. In addition, the rise of adjunctive biologic antibodies for asthmatic treatment has been witnessed, such as omalizumab, mepolizumab, and others. Even if a practitioner is not directly managing the patients' asthma care, this is a very exciting time for asthma diagnosis and treatment with advances in understanding, but it also serves as a reminder: While immunotherapy will likely help allergic asthma or asthma with T_h2 influences, it will not necessarily help all forms of asthma so be sure any asthmatic patient receiving immunotherapy understands that as well.

Clinical Pearls **M!**

- If you treat allergies, you're going to see patients with asthma.
- Be sure to assess known asthmatic patients' severity at initial visit.
- Be sure to assess known asthmatic patients' level of control at subsequent visits.
- Be suspicious of undiagnosed asthma in patients with complaints of coughing, wheezing, or similar symptoms.
- If you think the patient might have undiagnosed asthma, treat them like they do and send them for spirometry and/or pulmonary function testing. If you do not treat asthma, be sure to send them to a provider who does.

Bibliography

[1] Brożek JL, Bousquet J, Agache I, et al. Allergic Rhinitis and its Impact on Asthma (ARIA) guidelines-2016 revision. J Allergy Clin Immunol. 2017; 140(4):950–958

[2] National Heart, Lung, and Blood Institute. Asthma Quick Reference Guide. Available at https://www.nhlbi.nih.gov/files/docs/guidelines/asthma_qrg.pdf. Accessed May 22, 2019

[3] National Heart, Lung, and Blood Institute. Expert Panel Report 3 (EPR 3). Guidelines for the Diagnosis and Management of Asthma. Available at http://www.nhlbi.nih.gov/guidelines/asthma/asthgdln.htm. Accessed May 22, 2019

38 Food Allergy

Elizabeth J. Mahoney Davis, Matthew W. Ryan, Cecelia C. Damask

38.1 Food Allergy in a Nutshell

Food allergies are a growing health concern with a significant increase in reported prevalence. Allergic reactions to food can produce life-threatening anaphylaxis. Peanut allergy in particular is a significant public health problem. Peanut allergy often remains a life-long problem for many individuals, as less than 25% of peanut-allergic patients are expected to regain tolerance. Current recommendations for management include strict avoidance and a prescription for an auto-injectable form of epinephrine.

The increase in prevalence of peanut allergy occurred during a period of time when there was conflicting guidance regarding preventative measures for the development of peanut allergy. Before 2000, there were no guidelines regarding the timing for the introduction of peanut-containing products nor were there any purposeful strategies to delay the introduction of peanut-containing products to try to prevent the development of allergic disease. But in 2000, the American Academy of Pediatrics (AAP) recommended that "solid foods should not be introduced into the diet of high-risk infants until 6 months of age......and peanuts....until 3 years of age." This recommendation was reversed in 2008. At that time, AAP recommended that "the introduction of solid foods not be delayed past 4–6 months of age." However, they did not make any updated recommendations regarding the introduction of peanut-containing products.

The Learning Early About Peanut allergy (LEAP) study demonstrated that peanut-containing products can be safely introduced to high-risk infants between the ages of 4 and 11 months and that there is a monumental potential for peanut-allergy prevention. The National Institutes of Allergy and Infectious Diseases (NIAID) recently published an addendum guideline regarding the prevention of peanut allergy in the United States based on the findings from the LEAP study.

The NIAID-sponsored guidelines include the following three addendum recommendations:

1. Infants with severe eczema, egg allergy, or both should have introduction of age-appropriate peanut-containing food as early as 4 to 6 months of age to reduce the risk of peanut allergy. The Expert Panel recommended to strongly consider evaluation by in vitro specific immunoglobulin E (IgE) testing and/or skin prick testing (SPT), and if necessary an oral food challenge. Then based on these results, introduce peanut-containing foods.
2. Infants with mild-to-moderate eczema should have introduction of age-appropriate peanut-containing food around 6 months of age, in accordance with family preferences and cultural practices, to reduce the risk of peanut

allergy. The Expert Panel recommended that infants in this category may have dietary peanut introduced at home without an in-office evaluation. The Expert Panel recognized that some caregivers and health care providers may desire an in-office supervised feeding and/or evaluation.

3. Infants without eczema or any food allergy may have age-appropriate peanut-containing food freely introduced in their diet, together with other solid foods, and in accordance with family preferences and cultural practices.

There is an algorithm in the addendum guidelines to aid in assessing the high-risk infants in recommendation one. For these high-risk infants, it is recommended that they be evaluated and undergo skin testing by a specialist before the introduction of peanut-containing products. The Expert Panel did recognize that for those high-risk infants who do not have access to a specialist that testing for peanut-specific immunoglobulin E (sIgE) may be the preferred initial approach in certain instances.

The recommendations regarding when to introduce peanut-containing products into the diet have changed. New research demonstrated that early introduction of peanut-containing products around 4 to 6 months of age significantly reduced the risk of development of peanut allergy.

38.2 Definitions and Classification of Food Allergy

The first area of confusion when considering food allergy is its variable definition. A layperson may consider any adverse food reaction to be a "food allergy," while an allergist regards only a reaction with an immunologic mechanism to be a true food allergy. The 2010 Guidelines recommend that the term food allergy be used to describe an adverse health effect arising from a specific immune response that occurs reproducibly upon exposure to a given food. The guidelines further define food as any substance which is intended for human consumption including food additives, drinks, chewing gum, and dietary supplements. Food allergens are identified as the specific components of food (typically proteins but sometimes also chemical haptens) that are recognized by allergen-specific immune cells and elicit specific immunologic reactions resulting in characteristic symptoms. Patients can develop sensitization to food allergens without having clinical allergy symptoms. To be clear, patients may have detectable allergen-specific IgE to food allergens without having any clinical manifestations upon exposure to those same foods. The guidelines emphasize that sensitization alone is not sufficient to define food allergy. Finally, patients can have reproducible adverse reactions to specific foods that do not have an immunologic mechanism; these nonimmunologic reactions are defined as food intolerances and should not be confused with food allergy.

Many adverse reactions to food occur which may mimic food allergy but for which there is no immunologic basis. Such adverse food reactions, or food intolerances, include host-specific metabolic disorders such as galactosemia, alcohol intolerance, and lactose intolerance. Patients may also have reactions to a pharmacologically active component in a food, such as caffeine or tyramine in aged cheese. Additionally, individuals may react to toxic contaminants in food such as the histaminic chemical in the spoiled dark meat of certain fish, resulting in scombroid poisoning.

It is conceptually helpful for the clinician to categorize the broad spectrum of food-induced allergic disorders based on their underlying immunopathology. These categories of food allergy include: IgE-mediated, non-IgE-mediated, mixed IgE- and non-IgE-mediated, and cell-mediated.

IgE-mediated reactions are characterized by a temporal relationship between the reaction and exposure to the food. Most typically, symptoms of IgE-mediated food allergy occur within minutes to hours of exposure to the food. In the vast majority of these patients, serum food-specific IgE antibodies can be measured which, in conjunction with typical signs and symptoms on exposure to the food in question, confirm the IgE-mediated pattern of reaction. Just as with inhalant allergy, the diagnosis of allergy requires the presence of a positive patient history along with a positive test of IgE. A positive test (either in vitro IgE or skin prick test) alone does not translate to clinically relevant allergy.

Non-IgE-mediated immunologic reactions occur in some gastrointestinal disorders, particularly in children; these reactions are thought to be induced by delayed, immune but not IgE-mediated reactions to specific foods. Examples of these non-IgE-mediated reactions include food protein-induced enterocolitis syndrome, food protein-induced enteropathy syndrome, and food protein-induced allergic proctocolitis syndrome.

Mixed IgE- and non-IgE-mediated mechanisms should be considered when symptoms typically involving the gastrointestinal tract are of a more chronic nature and are not closely related to ingestion of the food. These syndromes include the eosinophilic gastroenteropathies: eosinophilic gastroenteritis, eosinophilic esophagitis, and eosinophilic proctocolitis.

Finally, allergic-contact dermatitis is an example of a cell-mediated allergic mechanism. Allergic-contact dermatitis represents a cell-mediated allergic reaction to chemical haptens that are present in food, and may be seen in food handlers.

A clear understanding of these definitions and classification schemes is important as the clinician reads the medical literature, and more importantly, embarks upon evaluating the patient with possible food allergy. Familiarity with food allergy concepts is important for the otolaryngologist because many patients with upper airway inflammatory disease are atopic and are at increased risk for having concomitant food allergy. In order to provide comprehensive care of the allergic patient, some knowledge of basic definitions, categories of food allergy, and clinical manifestations, and facility with diagnostic testing and treatment strategies for food allergy are important.

38.3 Treatment

The mainstay of treatment of food allergy currently is avoidance and elimination of offending food(s) from the patient's diet. Epinephrine is the first-line treatment in all cases of anaphylaxis, including food-induced anaphylaxis. A written food allergy emergency action plan which specifies when to use auto-injector epinephrine should be provided to patients with food allergies. A discussion regarding potential hidden sources of offending food(s) should occur with the patient and/or caregiver.

Investigations into potential treatments for food allergy have shown promise. There have been studies investigating the use of oral immunotherapy (OIT), sublingual immunotherapy (SLIT), and epicutaneous immunotherapy (EPIT). Oral immunotherapy involves mixing the offending food into a vehicle and having the patient consume it in a sequential, incrementally progressive fashion until a maintenance dose is achieved. Adverse reactions have been common in the OIT protocols with discontinuation occurring secondary to gastrointestinal symptoms. Furthermore, the studies suggest that OIT induces a transient desensitization rather than long-term tolerance. The SLIT studies involve administration of the allergen in liquid form under the tongue. The few published studies on SLIT suggest fewer adverse reactions than OIT, but the effects on induced desensitization do not seem to be as great compared to OIT. Epicutaneous immunotherapy involves applying an antigen-containing patch to the skin. Recently a study evaluating the clinical, safety, and immunologic effects of EPIT for the treatment of peanut allergy has been completed and it concluded that EPIT for peanut was safe and associated with a modest treatment response after 52 weeks.

At the time of writing this chapter, there are two treatments for peanut allergy that are being investigated by the Food and Drug Administration (FDA) for approval. AR101 is an OIT protocol that starts with 1 mg and ends with a 300-mg daily maintenance dose. Viaskin Peanut delivers a daily dose of 250 µg dose of peanut protein delivered through EPIT. Both therapies hope to improve the threshold dose that would result in symptoms from accidental exposure in a peanut-allergic patient. Neither therapy achieved sustained unresponsiveness to peanut in their respective trials.

There have been investigations into adjunctive therapies with OIT. There have been studies suggesting that adjunctive omalizumab with OIT expedites time to desensitization by allowing patients to start at a higher initial dose of OIT, by decreasing the number of doses required to reach maintenance dose, and that desensitization is maintained even after discontinuation of omalizumab. Also an anti–interleukin (IL)-33 antibody (ANB020) completed a phase 2 placebo-controlled clinical trial determining safety, tolerability, and activity in adult patients with peanut allergy. The phase 1 study indicated that a single dose was sufficient to suppress IL-33 function for approximately 3 months after dosing.

Clinical Pearls　**M!**

- The prevalence of food allergy appears to be increasing.
- Food allergy is defined as an adverse health effect arising from a specific immune response that occurs reproducibly on exposure to a given food and must be distinguished from food intolerance.
- Food allergies can be categorized as IgE-mediated, non-IgE-mediated, mixed IgE- and non-IgE-mediated, and cell-mediated.
- Different foods appear to affect different age groups. Cow's milk, hen's eggs, peanuts, and tree nuts account for most food allergy in young children, while adults are more likely to have allergies to shellfish, peanut, tree nuts, and fish.
- Evidence-based diagnostic testing modalities include SPT, food-allergen specific serum-IgE testing (sIgE), and oral food challenge. Both SPT and sIgE testing only measure sensitization. The double-blind, placebo-controlled food challenge is the gold standard for the diagnosis of food allergy.
- Avoidance of the offending food is the mainstay of treatment for food allergy. Patient education and preparation for accidental exposure are important in caring for the food-allergic patient.

Bibliography

[1] Boyce JA, Assa'ad A, Burks AW, et al. NIAID-Sponsored Expert Panel. Guidelines for the diagnosis and management of food allergy in the United States: report of the NIAID-sponsored expert panel. J Allergy Clin Immunol. 2010; 126(6) Suppl:S1–S58

[2] Togias A, Cooper SF, Acebal ML, et al. Addendum guidelines for the prevention of peanut allergy in the United States: Report of the National Institute of Allergy and Infectious Diseases-sponsored expert panel. J Allergy Clin Immunol. 2017; 139(1):29–44

39 Eosinophilic Esophagitis (EoE)

Cecelia C. Damask, Michael J. Parker

39.1 Most Interesting Information

- This is a clinicopathological condition characterized by symptoms of esophageal dysfunction and dense esophageal epithelial eosinophilia (> 15 eosinophils per high-power field [eos/HPF]).
- It's an enigmatic disease that mechanically is defined as an antigen-driven condition limited to the esophagus. It is an eosinophil-predominant disorder with a T_h2-cytokine profile suggestive of other allergic disorders, such as allergic rhinitis, asthma, and atopic dermatitis.
- Eosinophils reside in most of the gastrointestinal mucosa; however, they are not present in the normal esophageal epithelia.
- Similar to the airway remodeling that can occur in chronic asthma, eosinophilic esophagitis (EoE) can result in increased subepithelial collagen deposition, angiogenesis, and smooth muscle hypertrophy. Complications can result in esophageal remodeling with strictures and food impactions.

39.2 What Do We Know?

- Eosinophilic esophagitis is an allergen-driven disease.
- The most common triggers for EoE are foods. This is especially true for milk, egg, soy, and wheat.
- T_h2 inflammation via cytokines predominates the pathogenesis of EoE.
- Skin prick testing may be useful in children with EoE, but does not routinely demonstrate triggering food allergens in adults.
- Oral immunotherapy to both foods and pollens may trigger EoE.

39.3 What Is Still Unknown at This Time?

- What is the best way to test for potential allergens that may be triggering EoE?
- Are there allergen-specific T-cells in the esophagus that could be potential targets for treatment?
- Can immunotherapy be a treatment option for EoE?
- Will targeted modulation of the immune system be a therapeutic treatment option for EoE in the near future?

39.4 Prevalence

Eosinophilic esophagitis is a chronic, immune/antigen-mediated esophageal disease characterized clinically by symptoms related to esophageal dysfunction and histologically by eosinophil-predominant inflammation. Eosinophilic esophagitis is defined as a clinicopathologic diagnosis characterized by a localized eosinophilic inflammation of the esophagus (with no other gastrointestinal involvement), symptoms of esophageal dysfunction, the presence of 15 or more eosinophils in the most severely involved HPF isolated to the esophagus, and failure to respond to adequate proton-pump inhibitor (PPI) therapy. The Updated Consensus Recommendations for Children and Adults stresses that EoE is a clinicopathologic disease; both features are needed to make a diagnosis of EoE.

Estimates suggest that in the United States there are about 40 to 90 cases of EoE per 100,000 persons. The pediatric incidence of EoE approximates 1 per 10,000 population. Eosinophilic esophagitis can affect patients of any age. There is suggestion of a bimodal peak age of onset. In children, there is no peak after infancy whereas in adults, the peak incidence is from 30 to 40 years of age.

There is a strong association of EoE with atopic diseases. Patients with EoE have a higher rate of atopy than the general population. Majority (50–80%) of patients with EoE have other associated atopic conditions such as asthma, atopic dermatitis, and allergic rhinitis. Eosinophilic esophagitis shares many common immunologic features with other atopic diseases. Besides local eosinophilia, EoE also demonstrates impaired barrier function with infiltration of T-helper type 2 cells, basophils, mast cells, and type 2 innate lymphoid cells.

39.5 Clinical Presentation

The symptoms of EoE can include epigastric pain and vomiting but may also resemble the symptoms of gastroesophageal reflux disease (GERD). However, obstructive symptoms, such as dysphagia and food impactions, are typical in EoE and not in GERD. The predominant presenting symptom of EoE varies by age. Young children are more likely to present with feeding difficulties, failure to thrive, and classic GERD symptoms (epigastric pain) whereas older children are more likely to present similar to adults with dysphagia-type complaints and possible food impactions. It may be difficult for a young child to vocalize that they are having difficulty swallowing. They may exhibit refusal behavior and prolonged chewing. Even an older school-aged child or teenager may not complain of outright dysphagia but may exhibit some compensatory behaviors including taking small bites, drinking after each bite, or avoiding problematic foods such as meat and bread.

Classic symptoms of EoE in adults include dysphagia for solids and food impactions. The dysphagia may be either intermittent or chronic and is present in 25 to 100% of adult patients with EoE. A variety of other symptoms are also encountered, some of which are uncommon and not widely recognized. Although the most common symptom in adults is dysphagia, it is important to note that nonspecific symptoms such as nausea, vomiting, and abdominal pain may be the only clinical manifestation of EoE in selected adults. Food impaction can also occur in adults with EoE. It can either precede the diagnosis of EoE or be an ongoing manifestation of the disease. Food impaction warranting endoscopic removal is encountered in 33 to 54% of adult patients with EoE.

39.6 Endoscopic Findings

A wide variety of endoscopic findings may be seen in patients with EoE. These findings include concentric rings (described as "trachealization of the esophagus"), longitudinal furrows, white exudates/plaques (often confused with candidiasis), strictures, narrow-caliber esophagus, furrows, and even a normal-appearing esophagus. However, these findings are neither sensitive nor specific for EoE. Up to one-third of patients with active EoE may have a normal appearing esophagus, especially in children. Biopsies should ideally be taken from multiple sites in the proximal and distal esophagus as well as intestinal biopsies to rule out other disorders. The histologic abnormalities in patients with EoE are variable and a patchy distribution of esophageal eosinophilia has been reported. This observation stresses the importance of obtaining multiple biopsies in patients suspected of having EoE. A greater number of biopsies maximize the diagnostic yield.

39.7 Management

Pharmacologic, dietary, and endoscopic treatments for EoE have been established. Consensus guidelines emphasize the role of topical corticosteroids, dietary restriction, and endoscopic dilatation in improving symptomatology and reducing histologic eosinophilic burden with the ideal endpoint being complete resolution of the latter. Treatment options include medical management, esophageal dilatation, and food elimination diets. Currently, the use of swallowed steroids ("wrong way" steroids) is the mainstay of drug-based therapy. The two most commonly used "wrong way" steroids include swallowed aerosolized fluticasone propionate and oral budesonide mixed with Splenda™ (also honey, applesauce, and agave nectar can be used) to make it viscous. There have been variable dosing regimens presented in the literature as well as variable frequency and duration of treatment proposed. Although an optimal dose has not been established, fluticasone is usually administered twice a day.

Budesonide is to be mixed with 0.5 to 1.0 teaspoon of sweetener once a day in patients under 10 years of age and twice a day in those over 10 years of age. The patient is to swallow and not inhale the medication. Patients are to remain *nil per os* for 30 minutes after administration of a topical steroid. However, neither topical steroid is approved by the U.S. Food and Drug Administration (FDA) for treatment of EoE. Both topical ("wrong way") fluticasone and budesonide have shown efficacy in controlled trials. Systemic steroids are also a treatment option if topical steroid therapy fails or if rapid control of symptoms is needed.

Eosinophilic esophagitis is often considered a non-immunoglobulin E (IgE)-mediated food allergen-driven hypersensitivity, although the exact mechanism is unclear. It has been shown in both children and adults that food is a key trigger for EoE. Dietary management offers the possibility of inducing and maintaining prolonged disease remission without the potential complications associated with pharmacologic therapy such as esophageal candidiasis, cataracts, and adrenal suppression. Several types of dietary therapy have been used for patients with EoE. All food can be restricted when using a total elimination diet with an amino acid-based formula. Trials with elemental diets demonstrated greater than 90% histologic remission rates. However, in practicality, this is very difficult in clinical practice as the amino acid-based formula is often unpalatable and requires placement of a nasogastric (NG) tube for administration. Because elemental diets are unappealing, selective foods can be eliminated either based on allergy testing or by simply removing the foods most likely known to cause EoE ("the usual suspects"–milk, soy, egg, peanut, wheat, fish, and meats). Studies have shown mixed results with allergy-testing directed diets with outcomes inferior to elemental diets. The fact that allergy testing did not consistently predict the food triggers for EoE led to the use of empiric diets. The classic six food elimination diet (SFED) removes milk, wheat, egg, soy, fish/shellfish, and peanuts/tree nuts. Studies have shown histologic remission generally in 60 to 80% of cases with SFED. Studies also looked at an empiric four food elimination diet that removed milk, grains, eggs, and legumes. These studies demonstrated a 54% remission rate.

Another option is periodic dilatation. It is important to remember that dilatation will not address the underlying inflammation. A recent meta-analysis showed improvement with dilatation in 75% of patients. Potential complications with dilatation include esophageal perforation and hemorrhage.

A phase II randomized, double-blind, placebo-controlled clinical trial was conducted to assess the clinical efficacy of dupilumab for relieving symptoms in adult patients with EoE. The trial did reveal that dupilumab improved dysphagia, esophageal eosinophil counts, and esophageal distensibility compared to placebo.

Clinical Pearls M!

- Eosinophilic esophagitis can present differently in children and adults.
- It is one of the leading causes of food impaction and dysphagia in adults and vague reflux-like symptoms in children.
- Symptoms in children include vomiting, abdominal pain, and feeding difficulties; adults are characterized by the stereotypical features of food impaction, dysphagia, and, in some circumstances, chest pain.
- Disease occurring primarily in white males with an overall incidence of 1 in 10,000.
- Endoscopic patterns of linear furrows, circular ridges/concentric rings, and more defined rings (trachealization); the presence of white micro-abscesses; and the complication of severe strictures in some patients, are all manifestations of EoE.
- It is a chronic inflammatory disease which is often food-triggered. Ongoing research holds promise for possible novel treatment options for patients suffering with EoE.

Bibliography

[1] Dellon ES, Gonsalves N, Hirano I, Furuta GT, Liacouras CA, Katzka DA, American College of Gastroenterology. ACG clinical guideline: evidenced based approach to the diagnosis and management of esophageal eosinophilia and eosinophilic esophagitis (EoE). Am J Gastroenterol. 2013; 108 (5):679–692, quiz 693

[2] Dellow ES, Liacouras CA, Molina-Infante J, et al. Updated International Consensus Diagnostic Criteria for Eosinophilic Esophagitis: Proceedings of the AGREE Conference. Gastroenterology. 2018; 155(4):1022–1033

[3] Liacouras CA, Furuta GT, Hirano I, et al. Eosinophilic esophagitis: updated consensus recommendations for children and adults. J Allergy Clin Immunol. 2011; 128(1):3–20.e6, quiz 21–22

[4] Liacouras CA, Spergel J, Gober LM, Clinical Presentation in Children. Eosinophilic esophagitis: clinical presentation in children. Gastroenterol Clin North Am. 2014; 43(2):219–229

[5] Lucendo AJ, Molina-Infante J, Arias Á, et al. Guidelines on eosinophilic esophagitis: evidence-based statements and recommendations for diagnosis and management in children and adults. United European Gastroenterol J. 2017; 5(3):335–358

40 Atopic Dermatitis

Cecelia C. Damask

40.1 More than Skin Deep

Atopic dermatitis (AD) is a common, chronic inflammatory skin disease. It often commences in infancy and can remain a life-long struggle for patients. About 20 to 30% of children and 7 to 10% of adults are affected by AD. Almost 50% of children with AD continue to have symptoms into adulthood. Adult onset AD is considered a distinct subtype of AD; these patients are at increased risk for systemic complications including inflammatory bowel disease and rheumatoid arthritis.

The etiology of AD is thought to be multifactorial; a combination of impaired barrier dysfunction, immune dysregulation, and environmental risk factors. The barrier defect can result in skin sensitization to allergens. It is debated as to whether this is an "outside-in" model or an "inside-out" model.

The outside-in hypothesis proposes that AD is the result of genetic mutations affecting the epidermal barrier. Mutations of the filaggrin (*FLG*) gene cause defective expression of filaggrin, a barrier protection protein, which is important for the structure of the epidermis. Filaggrin plays a key role in epidermal hydration and pH regulation. *FLG* mutations have been linked to more severe and persistent AD. The outside-in hypothesis maintains that epidermal barrier disruption and allergen/microbe penetration cause immune dysfunction.

Whereas the inside-out hypothesis proposes that AD is caused by an inflammatory process inhibiting epidermal differentiation. The skin barrier becomes compromised after elevated T_h2 and T_h22 cytokine expression (interleukin [IL]-4, IL-13, IL-31) lead to localized inflammation and activation of other immune cells. The inside-out hypothesis is supported by evidence of elevated T-cell numbers present in nonlesional skin of AD patients.

Just like asthma, AD is a heterogeneous disorder. There is more than one inflammatory pathway that is involved in its pathogenesis. It is important to remember that the epithelial, immune, and microbial abnormalities in AD extend well beyond the inflamed skin. Atopic dermatitis does have systemic aspects. It is definitely more than skin deep.

Further suggestion that AD is more than skin deep includes the fact that patients with AD have significantly higher immunoglobulin E (IgE) responses than any other allergic disease, including asthma, food allergy, allergic rhinitis, and allergic conjunctivitis. Penetration of allergens through a defective skin barrier containing high levels of thymic stromal lymphopoietin (TSLP), IL-33, and IL-25 creates an ideal environment for increased IgE production.

Atopic dermatitis is often seen in conjunction with various atopic and allergic comorbidities, including food allergy, allergic rhinoconjunctivitis, and asthma. Atopic dermatitis can have significant effects on quality of life. These patients are often absent more frequently from work and school than their peers; disrupting not only their lives but their families' lives as well. The patients with AD complain of a debilitating chronic itch and skin pain that can dramatically affect sleep and lead to an increase in depression and anxiety.

40.2 Skin Barrier Care and Repair Are Paramount

Emollients, hydration (frequent baths), and topical corticosteroids play an important role in skin barrier protection and anti-inflammatory repair, and are considered basic management of AD. The use of emollients reduces the amount of topical steroids needed. Emollients can also help to reduce itching. Hydration is paramount in AD treatment. Ideally bathing should be performed at least once a day with emollients placed immediately afterward to prevent overdrying.

Identification and control of triggers, such as allergens, irritants, infections, and behavioral factors are also important. Topical corticosteroids (TCSs) are very effective both for acute flare-ups and also as maintenance therapy. With an acute flare-up, a twice daily application of a TCS is recommended. This can then be tapered down to twice a week on "known hot spots" for proactive maintenance therapy. Remember to not use high potency TCSs on sensitive areas such as the face and neck.

Other topical anti-inflammatory treatments for AD include topical calcineurin inhibitors (TCI) such as pimecrolimus and tacrolimus. These are safe on sensitive areas such as the face and neck. Both pimecrolimus and tacrolimus can be used twice daily for acute flare-ups and then weaned to two to three times a week on "known hot spots" for proactive maintenance therapy.

Another choice for anti-inflammatory therapy is crisaborale, a topical phosphodiesterase (PDE) 4 inhibitor. It is an enzyme that regulates inflammation by reducing certain inflammatory mediators including tumor necrosis factor α, interferon gamma (IFNγ), IL-12, IL-17, and IL-23. Crisaborale can be applied twice daily and can be used on sensitive areas such as the face and neck.

Systemic therapy may be considered in step-up care for AD patients uncontrolled with topical therapy. When AD is severe and cannot be controlled with topical therapies, phototherapy with a narrow band ultraviolet-B (UV-B) can be considered in selected patient groups. Other systemic therapy includes methotrexate, azathioprine, and cyclosporine A. Systemic corticosteroids should only be used in the context of bridging to another steroid-sparing treatment because severe rebound flare-ups occur after use with systemic corticosteroids.

40.3 Future of Atopic Dermatitis Treatment

Biologics (monoclonal antibodies) have shown great promise in the management of moderate-to-severe AD. Just as with asthma, not all biologics will be equally effective in all the different subtypes of AD.

Dupilumab blocks the α subunit of IL-4 receptor α, thus effectively blocking both IL-4 and IL-13, both of which are key cytokines implicated in the development of AD. Dupilumab demonstrated strong efficacy and safety for treatment of moderate-to-severe AD in adults. At the time of writing this chapter, dupilumab has only been approved for use in patients aged 12 years and older with moderate to severe AD that is not well controlled with topical therapies (TCS/TCI). During the clinical trials for approval, patients on dupilumab had overall higher rates of conjunctivitis than placebo. Dupilumab is dosed in adults at 300 mg subcutaneously every 2 weeks after an initial loading dose in adults of 600 mg. There are ongoing and planned studies for use in children as young as 6 months of age.

Phase II clinical studies with tralokinumab and lebrikizumab, anti-IL-13 antibodies, have demonstrated clinical efficacy in treatment of AD. IL-31 has been implicated as a mediator of itch in AD patients. Nemolizumab, anti-IL-31 receptor A antibody, demonstrated decrease in pruritus in a phase II clinical trial. Treatments targeting IL-22 and Janus kinases are also in development.

Clinical Pearls M!

- The etiology of AD is multifactorial.
- AD is a heterogenous disorder.
- It is not "just" a skin condition; there are systemic manifestations.
- Just as with asthma, "one size" does not "fit all" in terms of treatment approach for AD.
- Emollients, hydration, and topical anti-inflammatories are basic management.
- Biologics (monoclonal antibodies) have shown great promise as treatment options.

There have been significant advances in the understanding and management of AD. Studies have demonstrated that even the normal-appearing skin in patients with AD may have subclinical inflammation with evidence of skin barrier dysfunction. The focus has also expanded to include potential systemic aspects of AD beyond just the skin. Atopic dermatitis is definitely more than "just a skin condition."

Bibliography

[1] Boguniewicz M, Alexis AF, Beck LA, et al. Expert perspectives on management of moderate-to-severe atopic dermatitis: A multidisciplinary consensus addressing current and merging therapies. J Allergy Clin Immunol Pract. 2017; 5(6):1519–1531

[2] Boguniewicz M, Fonacier L, Guttman-Yassky E, Ong PY, Silverberg J, Farrar JR. Atopic dermatitis yardstick: practical recommendations for an evolving therapeutic landscape. Ann Allergy Asthma Immunol. 2018; 120(1):10–22.e2

[3] Izadi N, Leung DYM. Clinical approach to the patient with refractory atopic dermatitis. Ann Allergy Asthma Immunol. 2018; 120(1):23–33.e1

[4] Peng W, Novak N. Pathogenesis of atopic dermatitis. Clin Exp Allergy. 2015; 45(3):566–574

Part 7

Practice Makes Perfect

7

41 Worksheets on Allergy Testing with Answers

Christine B. Franzese

This chapter contains worksheets with examples of test results from hypothetical patients, which are similar to what a practitioner might actually encounter in practice. There are examples of skin prick testing results, intradermal dilutional testing results, modified quantitative testing results, and specific IgE testing results. If a practitioner is new to the practice of allergy, he/she may find these worksheets very helpful in testing knowledge or practicing what have been learned so far. Each worksheet is accompanied by a corresponding answer sheet. Enjoy!

Prick Testing Practice Case #1

The following are skin prick testing results from a hypothetical patient. Decide if each control/test is positive or negative and if the controls have responded appropriately.

Controls	Wheal (in mm)	Result [+/−]
Positive	7	
Negative (50% glycerin)	0	

Antigen	Wheal (in mm)	Result [+/−]
Timothy	7	
Bermuda	0	
Johnson	5	
Oak	2	
Alder	0	
Cedar	10	
Sycamore	3	
Pigweed	4	
Lambs' quarters	6	
Ragweed	0	
Mugwort sage	5	
D. pteronyssinus	8	
D. farinae	1	
Cat	9	
Dog	4	
Cockroach	0	
Aspergillus	0	
Alternaria	3	
Mucor	7	
Rhizopus	4	

Prick Testing Practice Case #1 (Answers)

The following are skin prick testing results from a hypothetical patient. The controls have responded appropriately.

Controls	Wheal (in mm)	Result [+/−]
Positive	7	+
Negative (50% glycerin)	0	−

Antigen	Wheal (in mm)	Result [+/−]
Timothy	7	+
Bermuda	0	−
Johnson	5	+
Oak	2	−
Alder	0	−
Cedar	10	+
Sycamore	3	+
Pigweed	4	+
Lambs' quarters	6	+
Ragweed	0	−
Mugwort sage	5	+
D. pteronyssinus	8	+
D. farinae	1	−
Cat	9	+
Dog	4	+
Cockroach	0	−
Aspergillus	0	−
Alternaria	3	+
Mucor	7	+
Rhizopus	4	+

Prick Testing Case #2

The following are skin prick testing results from a hypothetical patient. Decide if each control/test is positive or negative and if the controls have responded appropriately.

Controls	Wheal (in mm)	Result [+/−]
Positive	8	
Negative (50% glycerin)	4	

Antigen	Wheal (in mm)	Result [+/−]
Timothy	2	
Bermuda	3	
Johnson	11	
Oak	4	
Alder	10	
Cedar	0	
Sycamore	5	
Pigweed	8	
Lambs' quarters	13	
Ragweed	0	
Mugwort sage	3	
D. pteronyssinus	8	
D. farinae	1	
Cat	9	
Dog	4	
Cockroach	3	
Aspergillus	0	
Alternaria	4	
Mucor	9	
Rhizopus	3	

Prick Testing Case #2 (Answers)

While both the positive and negative controls have responded and are positive, the testing is still valid. This is because the positive control is ≥ 3 mm than the negative control. However, because the negative control is positive, it means the threshold to determine that a test is positive and not just an artifact of skin irritation caused by glycerin has increased. When this occurs, a positive test needs to be at least ≥ 3 mm than the negative control, or in this case, ≥ 7 mm.

Controls	Wheal (in mm)	Result [+/−]
Positive	8	+
Negative (50% glycerin)	4	+

Antigen	Wheal (in mm)	Result [+/−]
Timothy	2	−
Bermuda	3	−
Johnson	11	+
Oak	4	−
Alder	10	+
Cedar	0	−
Sycamore	5	−
Pigweed	8	+
Lambs' quarters	13	+
Ragweed	0	−
Mugwort sage	3	−
D. pteronyssinus	8	+
D. farinae	1	−
Cat	9	+
Dog	4	−
Cockroach	3	−
Aspergillus	0	−
Alternaria	4	−
Mucor	9	+
Rhizopus	3	−

Intradermal Dilutional Testing Case

The following are intradermal dilutional testing (IDT) testing results from a hypothetical patient. Decide if each control/test is positive or negative, if the controls have responded appropriately, and determine what the endpoint is for each antigen.

	Positive control (Wheal in mm) = 9		Negative control (Wheal in mm) = 2		Glycerin #1 control (Wheal in mm) = 5		
Antigen	#6	#5	#4	#3	#2	#1	Endpoint
Timothy	5	6	7	10			
Bermuda	5	7	11				
Johnson	8	8	8	8	10		
Oak	5	5	6	6	7	10	
Elm	5	5	5	6	6		
Cypress	5	7	9				
Sycamore	5	5	8	10			
Ragweed	5	6	6	6	9	11	
Pigweed	6	9	11				
English plantain	4	6	6	6	6		
D. pteronyssinus	9	12					
D. farinae	5	5	6	7	7	9	
Cat	6	7	9				
Cockroach	6	8	9	12			
Alternaria	5	5	6	8	11		
Aspergillus	4	4	5	5	6		

Intradermal Dilutional Testing Case (Answers)

The controls have responded appropriately. Testing is valid. The endpoint is the first positive test result followed by a confirmatory wheal that is 2 mm or greater.

Positive control (Wheal in mm) = 9			Negative control (Wheal in mm) = 2			Glycerin #1 control (Wheal in mm) = 5	
Antigen	#6	#5	#4	#3	#2	#1	Endpoint
Timothy	5	6	7	10			4
Bermuda	5	7	11				5
Johnson	8	8	8	8	10		3
Oak	5	5	6	6	7	10	2
Elm	5	5	5	6	6		Negative
Cypress	5	7	9				5
Sycamore	5	5	8	10			4
Ragweed	5	6	6	6	9	11	2
Pigweed	6	9	11				5
English plantain	4	6	6	6	6		Negative
D. pteronyssinus	9	12					6
D. farinae	5	5	6	7	7	9	2
Cat	6	7	9				5
Cockroach	6	8	9	12			4
Alternaria	5	5	6	8	11		3
Aspergillus	4	4	5	5	6		Negative

Modified Quantitative Testing Case

The following are modified quantitative testing (MQT) results from a hypothetical patient. Decide if each control/test is positive or negative, if the controls have responded appropriately, and determine an endpoint for each antigen.

Controls	Wheal (in mm)	ID	Result [+/−]	
Positive	8	7		
Negative (50% glycerin)	0	0		

	Prick	ID #2	ID #5	
Antigen	Wheal (in mm)	Wheal (in mm)	Wheal (in mm)	Endpoint
Timothy	3	5		
Bermuda	2	8		
Johnson	10			
Oak	4		0	
Alder	11		7	
Cedar	0	7		
Sycamore	6		2	
Pigweed	7		9	
Lambs' quarters	12		8	
Ragweed	3		0	
D. pteronyssinus	9			
D. farinae	2	7		
Cat	11		5	
Dog	4		5	
Cockroach	0	6		
Aspergillus	0	5		
Alternaria	4		11	
Mucor	7		5	
Rhizopus	3		5	

Abbreviation: ID, intradermal.

Modified Quantitative Testing Case (Answers)

The controls have responded appropriately.

Controls	Wheal (in mm)	ID	Result [+/−]	
Positive	8	7	+	
Negative (50% glycerin)	0	0	−	

	Prick	ID #2	ID #5	
Antigen	Wheal (in mm)	Wheal (in mm)	Wheal (in mm)	Endpoint
Timothy	3	5		Negative
Bermuda	2	8		3
Johnson	10			6
Oak	4		0	4
Alder	11		7	5
Cedar	0	7		3
Sycamore	6		2	4
Pigweed	7		9	6
Lambs' quarters	5		8	5
Ragweed	3		0	4
D. pteronyssinus	9			6
D. farinae	2	7		3
Cat	11		5	4
Dog	4		5	4
Cockroach	0	6		Negative
Aspergillus	0	5		Negative
Alternaria	4		11	6
Mucor	7		5	4
Rhizopus	3		5	4

Abbreviation: ID, intradermal.

Specific Immunoglobulin E Testing Case

Below are the testing results of a hypothetical patient who has undergone specific immunoglobulin E (IgE) testing. If a practitioner chooses to create a vial mix prescription for a patient using endpoints, this worksheet will help practice doing that. However, an endpoint doesn't need to be established in order to start immunotherapy treatment on a patient.

Antigen	Class #	Endpoint
Timothy	5	6
Bermuda	0	Negative/no endpoint
Johnson	1	2
Bahia	2	3
Oak	4	5
Elm	0	Negative/no endpoint
Cypress	3	4
Sycamore	0	Negative/no endpoint
Ragweed	6	7
Pigweed	2	3
Sheep sorrel	1	2
English plantain	0	Negative/no endpoint
D. pteronyssinus	3	4
D. farinae	4	5
Cat	6	7
Cockroach	5	6
Alternaria	0	Negative/no endpoint
Aspergillus	0	Negative/no endpoint
Mucor	3	4

Specific Immunoglobulin E Testing Case (Answers)

Below are the testing results of a hypothetical patient who has undergone specific IgE testing. If you choose to create a vial mix prescription for a patient using endpoints, this worksheet will help you practice doing that. However, you do not need to establish an endpoint if you choose not to in order to start immunotherapy treatment on a patient.

Antigen	Class #	Endpoint
Timothy	5	6
Bermuda	0	Negative/no endpoint
Johnson	1	2
Bahia	2	3
Oak	4	5
Elm	0	Negative/no endpoint
Cypress	3	4
Sycamore	0	Negative/no endpoint
Ragweed	6	7
Pigweed	2	3
Sheep sorrel	1	2
English plantain	0	Negative/no endpoint
D. pteronyssinus	3	4
D. farinae	4	5
Cat	6	7
Cockroach	5	6
Alternaria	0	Negative/no endpoint
Aspergillus	0	Negative/no endpoint
Mucor	3	4

42 Worksheets on Vial Mixing/Preparation with Answers

Christine B. Franzese

This chapter contains worksheets with examples of vial mixing prescriptions using testing results from hypothetical patients, which are similar to what a practitioner might actually encounter in practice. There are examples of 5 mL vials created for subcutaneous immunotherapy (SCIT), vials created for sublingual immunotherapy (SLIT), and an oral mucosal immunotherapy (OMIT) example. If a practitioner is new to the practice of allergy, he/she may find these worksheets very helpful in testing knowledge or practicing what have been learned so far. Each worksheet is accompanied by a corresponding answer sheet. Enjoy!

> For SCIT, some practitioners will determine an endpoint and some will not. An endpoint is not necessary to initiate SCIT or create a vial prescription. However, these worksheets can provide some practice for those who do like to or are interested in learning about endpoints.

Intradermal Dilutional Testing Vial Mixing Case Version 1

Below are the IDT testing results of a hypothetical patient. Determine an endpoint, and then using that endpoint, create a 5-mL vial mix prescription for the patient's first injection vial for SCIT. In this version, 50% glycerin is used to maintain the potency of vial as (PNS) is being used as the diluent.

Positive control
(Wheal in mm) = 9

Negative control
(Wheal in mm) = 2

Glycerin #1 control
(Wheal in mm) = 5

Vial prescription

Antigen	#6	#5	#4	#3	#2	#1	Endpoint
Timothy	5	6	7	10			
Bermuda	5	7	11				
Johnson	8	8	8	8	10		
Bahia	7	9					
Oak	5	5	6	6	7	10	
Elm	5	5	5	6	6		
Cypress	5	7	9				
Sycamore	5	5	8	10			
Ragweed	5	6	6	6	9	11	

Dilution #	Volume
Total antigen	
50% glycerin	
Diluent	
Total	

Intradermal Dilutional Testing Vial Mixing Case Version 1 (Answers)

Below are the answers for the IDT testing results of a hypothetical patient, including the endpoints and starting dilutions for the patient's first injection vial for SCIT. This vial is 5 mL in size, but similar math could be used to create a 10-mL vial. In this version, 50% glycerin is used to maintain the potency of vial as PNS is being used as the diluent. In order to maintain potency, the vial must contain at least 1 mL of 50% glycerin.

Positive control
(Wheal in mm) = 9

Negative control
(Wheal in mm) = 2

Glycerin #1 control
(Wheal in mm) = 5

Vial prescription

Antigen	#6	#5	#4	#3	#2	#1	Endpoint
Timothy	5	6	7	10			4
Bermuda	5	7	11				5
Johnson	8	8	8	8	10		3
Bahia	7	9					6
Oak	5	5	6	7	10		3
Elm	5	5	5	6	6		Negative
Cypress	5	7	9				5
Sycamore	5	5	8	10			4
Ragweed	5	6	6	9	11		3

Dilution #	Volume
2	0.2 mL
3	0.2 mL
1	0.2 mL
4	0.2 mL
1	0.2 mL
3	0.2 mL
2	0.2 mL
1	0.2 mL
Total antigen	0.8 mL
50% glycerin	1.0 mL
Diluent	3.2 mL
Total	5.0 mL

229

Intradermal Dilutional Testing Vial Mixing Case Version 2

▶ Table 42.1 shows the IDT testing results of a hypothetical patient. Determine an endpoint, and then using that endpoint, create a 5-mL vial mix prescription for the patient's first injection vial for SCIT. In this version, HSA is used as the diluent to maintain potency of the vial.

	Positive control (Wheal in mm) = 9				Negative control (Wheal in mm) = 2			Glycerin #1 control (Wheal in mm) = 5	

Vial prescription

Antigen	#6	#5	#4	#3	#2	#1	Endpoint	Dilution #	Volume
Pigweed	6	9	11						
Sheep sorrel	5	9	9	9	12				
English plantain	4	6	6	6	6				
D. pteronyssinus	9	12							
D. farinae	5	5	6	7	7	9			
Cat	6	7	9						
Cockroach	6	8	9	12					
Alternaria	5	5	6	8	11				
Aspergillus	4	4	5	5	6				
Mucor	8	11							

Total antigen	
50% glycerin	
Diluent	
Total	

Intradermal Dilutional Testing Vial Mixing Case Version 2 (Answers)

Below are the answers for the IDT testing results of a hypothetical patient, including the endpoints and starting dilutions for the patient's first injection vial for SCIT. In this example a 5-mL vial is made, but similar math could be used to create a 10-mL vial. In this version, HSA is used as the diluent to maintain potency of the vial. It is not necessary to add glycerin when using HSA.

C=Concentrate (antigen concentrate)

Positive control (Wheal in mm) = 9	Negative control (Wheal in mm) = 2	Glycerin #1 control (Wheal in mm) = 5

Vial prescription

Antigen	#6	#5	#4	#3	#2	#1	Endpoint		Dilution #	Volume
Pigweed	6	9	11				5		3	0.2 mL
Sheep sorrel	5	9	9	9	12		3		1	0.2 mL
English plantain	4	6	6	6	6		Negative			
D. pteronyssinus	9	12					6		4	0.2 mL
D. farinae	5	5	6	7	7	9	2		C	0.2 mL
Cat	6	7	9				5		3	0.2 mL
Cockroach	6	8	9	12			4		2	0.2 mL
Alternaria	5	5	6	8	11		3		1	0.2 mL
Aspergillus	4	4	5	5	6		Negative			
Mucor	8	11					6		4	0.2 mL
									Total antigen	1.4 mL
									50% glycerin	NONE
									Diluent (HSA)	3.6 mL
									Total	5.0 mL

Vial Mixing Escalation Case Version 1

Below are the intradermal dilutional testing (IDT) endpoint results of a hypothetical patient. Create a 5-mL vial mix prescription for the patient's first injection vial for SCIT, then the subsequent two escalation vials. In this version, 50% glycerin is used to maintain the potency of vial as phenolated normal saline (PNS) is being used as a diluent.

1st Escalation vial

Antigen	Endpoint	Dilution #	Volume
Timothy	6		
Johnson	4		
Maple	3		
Oak	5		
Cypress	4		
Ragweed	6		
Sheep sorrel	3		
D. pteronyssinus	6		
D. farinae	5		
Dog	6		
Cockroach	6		
		Total antigen	
		50% glycerin	
		Diluent	
		Total	

2nd Escalation vial

Dilution #	Volume
Total antigen	
50% glycerin	
Diluent	
Total	

3rd Escalation vial

Dilution #	Volume
Total antigen	
50% glycerin	
Diluent	
Total	

Vial Mixing Escalation Case Version 1 (Answers)

Below are the IDT endpoint results of a hypothetical patient. Create a 5-mL vial mix prescription for the patient's first injection vial for SCIT, then the subsequent two escalation vials. In this version, 50% glycerin is used to maintain the potency of vial as PNS is being used as a diluent. Conc=concentrate.

		1st Escalation vial		2nd Escalation vial		3rd Escalation vial	
Antigen	Endpoint	Dilution #	Volume	Dilution #	Volume	Dilution #	Volume
Timothy	6	4	0.2 mL	3	0.2 mL	2	0.2 mL
Johnson	4	2	0.2 mL	1	0.2 mL	Conc	0.2 mL
Maple	3	1	0.2 mL	Conc	0.2 mL	Conc	0.2 mL
Oak	5	3	0.2 mL	2	0.2 mL	1	0.2 mL
Cypress	4	2	0.2 mL	1	0.2 mL	Conc	0.2 mL
Ragweed	6	4	0.2 mL	3	0.2 mL	2	0.2 mL
Sheep sorrel	3	1	0.2 mL	Conc	0.2 mL	Conc	0.2 mL
D. pteronyssinus	6	4	0.2 mL	3	0.2 mL	2	0.2 mL
D. farinae	5	3	0.2 mL	2	0.2 mL	1	0.2 mL
Dog	6	4	0.2 mL	3	0.2 mL	2	0.2 mL
Cockroach	6	4	0.2 mL	3	0.2 mL	2	0.2 mL
Total antigen			2.2 mL	Total antigen	2.2 mL	Total antigen	2.2 mL
50% glycerin			1 mL	50% glycerin	0.6 mL	50% glycerin	0.2 mL
Diluent			1.8 mL	Diluent	2.2 mL	Diluent	2.6 mL
Total			5.0 mL	Total	5.0 mL	Total	5.0 mL

Vial Mixing Escalation Case Version 2

Below are the IDT endpoint results of a hypothetical patient. Create a 5-mL vial mix prescription for the patient's first injection vial for SCIT, then the subsequent two escalation vials. In this version, human serum albumen (HSA) is used as the diluent to maintain the potency of vial.

1st Escalation vial

Antigen	Endpoint	Dilution #	Volume
Timothy	6		
Johnson	4		
Maple	3		
Oak	5		
Cypress	4		
Ragweed	6		
Sheep sorrel	3		
D. pteronyssinus	6		
D. farinae	5		
Dog	6		
Cockroach	6		
		Total antigen	
		Diluent	
		Total	

2nd Escalation vial

Dilution #	Volume
Total antigen	
Diluent	
Total	

3rd Escalation vial

Dilution #	Volume
Total antigen	
Diluent	
Total	

Vial Mixing Escalation Case Version 2 (Answers)

Below are the IDT endpoint results of a hypothetical patient. Create a 5-mL vial mix prescription for the patient's first injection vial for SCIT, then the subsequent two escalation vials. In this version, HSA is used as the diluent to maintain the potency of vial. Conc=concentrate

1st Escalation vial

Antigen	Endpoint	Dilution #	Volume
Timothy	6	4	0.2 mL
Johnson	4	2	0.2 mL
Maple	3	3	0.2 mL
Oak	5	3	0.2 mL
Cypress	4	2	0.2 mL
Ragweed	6	4	0.2 mL
Sheep sorrel	3	3	0.2 mL
D. pteronyssinus	6	4	0.2 mL
D. farinae	5	3	0.2 mL
Dog	6	4	0.2 mL
Cockroach	6	4	0.2 mL
		Total antigen	2.2 mL
		Diluent	2.8 mL
		Total	5.0 mL

2nd Escalation vial

Dilution #	Volume
3	0.2 mL
3	0.2 mL
Conc	0.2 mL
2	0.2 mL
3	0.2 mL
3	0.2 mL
Conc	0.2 mL
3	0.2 mL
2	0.2 mL
3	0.2 mL
3	0.2 mL
Total antigen	2.2 mL
Diluent	2.8 mL
Total	5.0 mL

3rd Escalation vial

Dilution #	Volume
2	0.2 mL
Conc	0.2 mL
Conc	0.2 mL
3	0.2 mL
Conc	0.2 mL
2	0.2 mL
Conc	0.2 mL
2	0.2 mL
3	0.2 mL
2	0.2 mL
2	0.2 mL
Total antigen	2.2 mL
Diluent	2.8 mL
Total	5.0 mL

Sublingual Immunotherapy Vial Mixing Case

Below are the skin prick test (SPT) results for a hypothetical patient interested in SLIT drops. This worksheet will help in making the maintenance and only one escalation vial. Remember the difference in vial size. Most SLIT vials are larger than SCIT vials.

		Maintenance vial		Escalation vial	
Antigen	**SPT result**	**Dilution #**	**Volume**	**Dilution #**	**Volume**
Timothy	6			Maintenance vial	
Johnson	4			50% glycerin	
Oak	5			Total	
Cypress	4				
Ragweed	6				
D. pteronyssinus	6				
D. farinae	5				
Cat	6				
		Total antigen			
		50% glycerin			
		Total			

Sublingual Immunotherapy Vial Mixing Case (Answers)

Below are the SPT results for a hypothetical patient interested in SLIT drops. This worksheet will help in making the maintenance and only one escalation vial. Remember the difference in vial size. Most SLIT vials are larger than SCIT vials. Conc=Concentrate

Maintenance vial

Antigen	SPT result	Dilution #	Volume
Timothy	6	Conc	1.0 mL
Johnson	4	Conc	1.0 mL
Oak	5	Conc	1.0 mL
Cypress	4	Conc	1.0 mL
Ragweed	6	Conc	1.0 mL
D. pteronyssinus	6	Conc	1.0 mL
D. farinae	5	Conc	1.0 mL
Cat	6	Conc	1.0 mL
		Total antigen	8.0 mL
		50% glycerin	2.0 mL
		Total	10.0 mL

Escalation vial

Dilution #	Volume
Maintenance vial	0.25 mL
50% glycerin	1.0 mL
Total	1.25 mL

Specific Immunoglobulin E Vial Mixing Case

Below are the testing results of a hypothetical patient who has undergone specific immunoglobulin E (IgE) testing. Create a vial mix prescription for this patient using endpoints. In this scenario, practice making two versions of the same vial, one with glycerin as the preservative and another using HSA.

Antigen	Class #	Endpoint	Vial using glycerin		Vial using HSA	
			Dilution #	Volume	Dilution #	Volume
Timothy	5					
Bermuda	0					
Bahia	2					
Oak	0					
Elm	0					
Cypress	3					
Ragweed	6					
Sheep sorrel	1					
English plantain	0					
D. pteronyssinus	3					
D. farinae	0					
Cat	0					
Cockroach	5					
Alternaria	0					
Aspergillus	0					
Mucor	3					
			Total antigen		Total antigen	
			50% glycerin		Diluent	
			Diluent		Total	
			Total			

Specific Immunoglobulin E Vial Mixing Case (Answers)

Below are the testing results of a hypothetical patient who has undergone specific IgE testing. Create a vial mix prescription for this patient using endpoints. In this scenario, practice making two versions of the same vial, one with glycerin as the preservative and another using HSA.

Antigen	Class #	Endpoint	Vial using glycerin		Vial using HSA	
			Dilution #	Volume	Dilution #	Volume
Timothy	5	6	4	0.2 mL	4	0.2 mL
Bermuda	0					
Bahia	2	3	1	0.2 mL	1	0.2 mL
Oak	0					
Elm	0					
Cypress	3	4	2	0.2 mL	2	0.2 mL
Ragweed	6	7	5	0.2 mL	5	0.2 mL
Sheep sorrel	1	2	Conc	0.2 mL	Conc	0.2 mL
English plantain	0					
D. pteronyssinus	3	4	2	0.2 mL	2	0.2 mL
D. farinae	0					
Cat	0					
Cockroach	5	6	4	0.2 mL	4	0.2 mL
Alternaria	0					
Aspergillus	0					
Mucor	3	4	2	0.2 mL	2	0.2 mL
			Total antigen	1.6 mL	Total antigen	1.6 mL
			50% glycerin	0.8 mL	Diluent	3.4 mL
			Diluent	2.6 mL	Total	5.0 mL
			Total	5.0 mL		

Oral Mucosal Immunotherapy Mixing Case

Below are the skin prick test (SPT) results for a hypothetical patient interested in OMIT. This worksheet will in making the OMIT prescription.

OMIT recipe

Antigen	SPT result	Dilution #	Volume
Bermuda	6		
Johnson	4		
Birch	5		
Sycamore	4		
Ragweed	6		
D. pteronyssinus	6		
D. farinae	5		
Aspergillus	6		
		Total antigen	
		50% glycerin	
		Total	

Oral Mucosal Immunotherapy Mixing Case (Answers)

Below are the skin prick test (SPT) results for a hypothetical patient interested in OMIT. This worksheet will help in making the OMIT prescription.

OMIT recipe

Antigen	SPT result	Dilution #	Volume
Bermuda	6	Conc	2.0 mL
Johnson	4	Conc	2.0 mL
Birch	5	Conc	2.0 mL
Sycamore	4	Conc	2.0 mL
Ragweed	6	Conc	2.0 mL
D. pteronyssinus	6	Conc	2.0 mL
D. farinae	5	Conc	2.0 mL
Aspergillus	6	Conc	2.0 mL
		Total antigen	16.0 mL
		50% glycerin	4.0 mL
		Total	20.0 mL

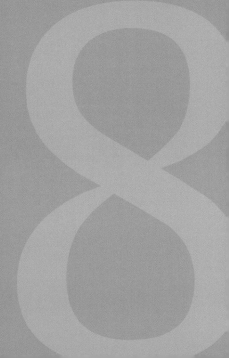

Part 8

Adding Allergy to Your Practice

43 USP <797> and Compounding

Cecelia C. Damask, Christine B. Franzese

43.1 What Is USP Chapter <797>?

Understanding the risks inherent in sterile compounding and incorporating established standards are essential for patient safety. Compounded drugs made without the guidance of standards may be subpotent, superpotent, or contaminated, exposing patients to significant risk of adverse events or even death.

United States Pharmacopeia (USP) develops standards for preparing compounded sterile drugs to help ensure patient benefit and reduce risks such as contamination, infection, or incorrect dosing.

USP General Chapter <797> describes a number of requirements, including responsibilities of compounding personnel, training, facilities, environmental monitoring, and storage and testing of finished preparations.

43.2 What Is Next Iteration of the USP Chapter <797> Draft?

In September 2015, the USP released a proposed updated Chapter 797 on procedures for sterile compounding. The existing chapter had provided procedures for allergen immunotherapy extracts as a separate element to processes applicable to three levels of risk for other sterile compounded products. The September 2015 draft collapsed those requirements into just two categories; treating all sterile compounds, including allergen extract, as equally and inherently dangerous. At the time of the writing of this chapter, the updated draft was open for public comment. The anticipated official date for < 797 > to go into effect will be December 1, 2019.

Allergen extract is restored as a separate section of the proposed draft chapter. The allergen extract compounding requirements address compounding personnel training and evaluation, hygiene and garbing, and updated documentation requirements, plus either installation of an ISO Class 5, Primary Engineering Control (PEC), *or* a dedicated Allergenic Extracts Compounding Area (AECA), with specifications and requirements provided for either option.

43.3 Who Does the Mixing?

The preparation of compounded sterile preparations (CSPs) is defined as combining, admixing, diluting, pooling, reconstituting, repackaging, or otherwise altering a drug or bulk drug substance to create a sterile medication. There are minimum requirements that apply to all persons who prepare CSPs. This includes, but is not limited to, pharmacists, technicians, physicians, and nurses in all places including, but not limited to, hospitals and other health care institutions, patient treatment sites, infusion facilities, pharmacies, and physicians' or practice sites.

Compounding staff will be required to be trained and regularly evaluated on aseptic and compounding technique, mostly reflecting existing requirements but with the addition of gloved fingertip testing and thumb sampling and appropriate incubation of samples to ensure proper sterile technique is being followed. These requirements will help maintain consistent attention to the foremost importance of ensuring patient safety. Documentation requirements for compounding procedures, temperature logs for refrigeration, and prescription set documentation reflect best practices.

43.4 Where Does the Mixing Occur?

With the establishment of a dedicated AECA, including requirements for the surfaces and surrounding area, a hood is *not* required. The requirements for an AECA include no carpeting, impervious surfaces, no outside doors or openable windows, a visible perimeter, and additional reasonable expectations for sterile compounding in the physician's office.

43.5 What Is Aseptic Compounding Technique?

Aseptic compounding technique is preparing materials to be compounded in a sterile fashion in a specific site (AECA), where the surface preparation area has been sanitized with 70% isopropanol that does not contain added ingredients, such as dyes and glycerin. Compounding personnel must thoroughly wash and remove debris from under fingernails (using a nail cleaner under running warm water), followed by vigorous hand and arm washing to the elbows for at least 30 seconds with either nonantimicrobial or antimicrobial soap or perform antiseptic hand cleansing with an alcohol-based surgical hand scrub with persistent activity or both, before beginning any compounding. They must also wear hair covers, facial hair covers, gowns, face masks, and powder-free sterile gloves that are compatible with sterile 70% isopropyl alcohol. All vial stoppers and any necks of ampules to be opened must be sanitized with 70% isopropyl alcohol and confirmed that the critical sites are wet for at least 10 seconds and allowed to dry before they are used to compound. Avoid direct contamination of any sterile needles, syringes, or other devices. Gloves should be periodically disinfected with sterile 70% isopropyl alcohol when preparing multiple allergenic extract vials. After all mixing/compounding is complete, a visual inspection should be done to ensure the vial is intact and labeled appropriately.

43.6 How Is Aseptic Compounding Technique Measured?

One method to evaluate aseptic compounding technique is an annual technical drill called a media-fill test and it is recommended that all individuals who prepare extract vials pass such a test. This tests the performance of compounding personnel's aseptic technique using a sterile microbiological growth medium, rather than allergy extract, to test whether the aseptic procedures are adequate to prevent contamination during actual allergen compounding. This type of test is available from several manufacturers as a kit to test one or more compounding personnel. Be sure to follow the manufacturer's instructions/recommendations for the test you purchase.

43.7 What Is Gloved Fingertip and Thumb Testing and Why Is That Needed or Being Added?

Protected gowning and gloving, even when done properly, isn't 100% effective. When gowns or gloves are brushed or touched, they can cause inadvertent contamination in different ways, including a "bellows" effect that may cause shed skin cells and bacteria to become airborne contaminates. The amount of skin and bacteria shed by individuals is variable, and there are some individuals termed "shedders," who have higher than average rates of emitting skin debris and bacterial contaminants.

Gloved fingertip and thumb testing uses sterile petri plates to sample parts of compounding personnel's hands after protective garb has been donned. How frequently this must be done likely will depend on the level of risk associated with the type of compounding being done. Similar to the media-fill test, these types of tests are available from several manufacturers.

Clinical Pearls   M!

- Allergy involves compounding which falls under USP < 797 > requirements.
- These guidelines are currently undergoing revision, with the new chapter to be released in 2019.
- Compounding personnel need to be trained, garbed, and periodically evaluated on their aseptic techniques.
- While a hood does not seem to be required, ensure that the space were antigens are being compounded complies with the requirements for an AECA.

Bibliography

[1] The United States Pharmacopeial Convention. <797> Pharmaceutical Compounding—Sterile Pre-parations, Revision 2008. Available at https://www.sefh.es/fichadjuntos/USP797GC.pdf. Accessed September 1, 2018

[2] The United States Pharmacopeial Convention. DRAFT <797> Pharmaceutical Compounding—Sterile Preparations, Revision pending 2018. Available at http://www.usp.org/sites/default/files/usp/document/our-work/compounding/proposed-revisions-gc-797.pdf. Accessed September 1, 2018

44 Office Set-up

William R. Reisacher, Matthew W. Ryan, Cecelia C. Damask

44.1 Why Add Allergy to an Existing Practice?

There are many reasons why a practitioner may consider adding allergy to a practice:
- You may have always had an interest in allergies.
- You may be filling a need in your community.
- You may seek to provide comprehensive care for patients with aerodigestive tract inflammatory disease.

Whatever the reason or reasons may be for embarking on this journey, the prerequisites are believing that allergies have a significant impact on a patient's quality of life and having the commitment to deliver allergy care in a safe and effective manner. Many of the patients who come into the office have allergies contributing in some way to their chief complaint, and in truth, allergy is already being practiced in most providers' offices, whether he/she realizes it or not.

44.2 What Exactly Does It Mean to "Add Allergy" to the Office?

This may mean something different for each practice. Allergic disease can be diagnosed and treated without adding a single element to the office. A good history and physical examination can detect allergic disease and environmental control strategies can be discussed from that point. Medical trials can be initiated and adjusted based on symptomatic relief and this approach has proven to be very successful for many patients. "Adding allergy" to a practice really means that the clinician would like to confirm the presumptive diagnosis of allergy, identify suspected allergens through specific testing, and provide allergen-specific immunotherapy to those patients whose quality of life suffers despite pharmacotherapy and avoidance strategies.

When it comes to adding allergy to your practice, one size definitely does not fit all. Through time, each physician must learn how allergy works best in their particular situation. It is inevitable that many obstacles will be encountered, but if the physician is prepared to start slow, ask many questions, and always keep the welfare of their patients as the top priority, then the decision to add allergy to the practice will be a rewarding one for both doctor and patient.

44.3 Factors to Consider

If a practitioner is contemplating adding allergy to the practice, he/she must first consider the impact an allergy service would have on the practice. A practitioner may have decided that adding allergy is the best move for the practice, but the other partners in the practice may not necessarily be in agreement. Some partners may be concerned about a shift in the patient mix or the way such a change will be perceived by the community. If the practice is currently referring to other allergists in the community, adding allergy to the practice might affect the referrals coming from those sources, and these issues must be considered and thoroughly discussed before moving forward.

Another factor to consider is whether an allergy service is financially feasible for the practice at the moment. This is another area where the partners must all be in agreement, particularly when each member will be sharing the financial burden. There are significant start-up costs, and this chapter will help you understand all the elements that go into calculating this. Eventually, an allergy service will become a source of revenue for the practice, but this may take time depending on the situation. If the allergy service becomes busy quickly, start-up costs may be recovered in the first 6 months. But if there aren't many practitioners referring allergy patients at first, it may take a year or even longer.

Once there is general agreement within the practice to add allergy, the next step is to look around the community and see how, where, and by whom allergy care is currently being provided. If there is a large general allergy practice down the road, or a nearby ENT practice that provides allergy services, you may encounter some difficulties in recruiting patients. However, if established offices are only able to offer new appointments in 3 months, a new allergy service may attract a great deal of business.

Fortunately, you can acquire a large number of allergy patients from your own practice. Ultimately, you must decide when and how aggressively to start advertising the new allergy service. Giving talks to other practices, schools, and community groups can be helpful in getting the word out and will also educate others about newer techniques, such as sublingual immunotherapy (SLIT) or possibly even oral mucosal immunotherapy (OMIT).

Once word spreads in the community about the new allergy practice, there may be some negative feedback. Some may respond to this medical and financial threat to their territory with statements that are unkind or simply untrue. In these unfortunate situations, you must stay focused on patient care rather than resorting to similar tactics. Satisfied patients speak loudly enough.

It may be useful to reach out to others during this part of the process. Talking to established allergists may provide new ideas on how to proceed and advice on how to avoid common pitfalls. If possible, a visit to one or two other offices that provide allergy services for a day of observation may provide even further inspiration. It is also helpful to talk to practice consultants who can estimate the financial ability of the practice to add allergy, estimate the necessary changes in staff and educate the physician about the current allergy codes and billing practices. Speaking to the practice lawyer is also useful to assure that there will be no legal ramifications of adding allergy to the practice, such as a restrictive clause in the lease prohibiting that type of practice in the building, and that it is considered within your scope of practice.

There also tends to be a shift in the patient mix and practitioner and their partners must be willing to accept this. Once allergy is added to the practice, there will invariably be a shift toward allergy and sinus patients, possibly at the expense of other types of patients. There may also be a shift in the surgical caseload, both in type and volume, if there are surgical providers in the practice. A practitioner may also start seeing patients with problems that are indirectly related to allergies, such as asthma and dermatitis. Each provider must decide where their comfort level is in evaluating these conditions and decide to refer to others or obtain additional training when necessary. A practitioner must also be prepared to make referrals to dermatologists or pulmonologists when appropriate.

44.4 Preparing the Office

44.4.1 Allergy Training

After making the decision to proceed with adding allergy to the practice, the next choice is whether the practitioner will be going to lead this service or hire someone else. This could include a general allergist or another physician who has allergy training. However, consideration should be given to whether or not the practice has reached the point where it can support another provider, particularly if that individual is not able to bring established patients right into the practice. Regardless of who is providing allergy services, when allergy testing and immunotherapy are taking place in the office, all physicians and staff members must be educated about recognizing the signs of anaphylaxis and a protocol must be in place to treat this emergency.

44.4.2 Which Services to Offer

In laying the foundation for the allergy service, a practitioner must decide whether to use exclusive serum-specific immunoglobulin E (IgE) testing (in vitro) or a combination of skin and in vitro testing. In vitro testing may be performed in the office, but this service is under strict regulation by the Clinical Laboratory Improvement Amendments (CLIA) of 1988, and special certification is required. For this reason, most send in vitro testing to reference laboratories and receive the results in less than a week. In vitro testing should be available for those patients who cannot or should not be skin tested, such as histamine nonreactors, those with dermatographia, very young children, and pregnant women. Panels for in vitro testing should be chosen as judiciously as those for skin testing.

A practitioner may choose to perform skin testing in allergy practices. This was discussed in detail in previous chapters, but usually involves skin prick testing (SPT), intradermal testing (IDT), or a combination of both, such as modified quantitative testing (MQT). Performing skin testing in the office naturally involves more training, office space, and lab personnel than in vitro testing. A practitioner may choose to use one method exclusively for testing, either a type of skin testing or in vitro testing, or may use both. Regardless of the chosen method, the best advice is to be safe, consistent, and always use clinical suspicion to guide testing.

Other skin testing which may be offered might include specific testing for penicillin allergy, which is now commercially available, or patch testing. Patch testing, which is most commonly performed by dermatologists, is used for chemicals and substances that may contact the skin and produce a delayed (type IV) reaction.

Another service that may be considered for the new allergy patients is pulmonary function testing (PFT). Pulmonary function testing is very useful when the practitioner is providing asthma medications. Pulmonary function testing changes may help the practitioner decide whether or not seasonal asthmatics should be tested or receive an immunotherapy injection, and may also be used to document their progress after a course of medication or immunotherapy. Small, portable PFT units are available which may be linked to a computer or network so results appear immediately in the patient's chart. Testing may also be performed before and after inhalation of a short-acting beta agonist to demonstrate the reversibility of airway obstruction—a hallmark of asthma. Again, a practitioner must decide which asthma patients he/she is comfortable treating and recognize the right time to consult with a pulmonologist.

Immunotherapy, also known as desensitization, is a common service provided; usually reserved for allergic patients whose symptoms or comorbidities have not been adequately relieved with pharmacotherapy and environmental control strategies. Since it was introduced by Noon in 1911, subcutaneous immunotherapy (SCIT) has been administered through the injection route. But since the 1960s, sublingual immunotherapy (SLIT) has also been available using liquid extract drops. While adding allergy to the practice, a practitioner must decide whether to use one or more of these methods. While both methods have been found to be similar in terms of efficacy, SCIT is generally performed weekly in the office and is covered by most insurance plans, while SLIT is administered daily at home and is not covered by insurance. There are also FDA-approved SLIT tablets available for daily use at home. Each of these methods of immunotherapy can be started based on in vitro or skin testing.

If a practitioner is going to provide immunotherapy services, he/she must decide whether to formulate and prepare the vials in the office or have this done by an outside source. Outsourcing this service is useful if space and resources in the office are limited, but disadvantages include the loss of individualized control of the vials, the loss of revenue for this service, and the fact that the treating extract may differ from the testing extract. After the patient is tested, the practitioner decides which allergens should be included in the vial and the level of sensitivity to those allergens. Once the outside company returns the vials, an intradermal vial test is performed for SCIT vials to ensure safety and injections are begun. Treatment with SLIT drops or tablets may also be performed in a similar fashion, with the first dose administered in the office.

44.4.3 Preparing Space for Allergy

The decision to add allergy to the practice will also lead to some physical changes in the office. The amount of space required for the new allergy service will be dictated by the types of services being offered as well as financial limitations, but the first question is whether to use existing space or add a new space. Adding a new space could mean minor renovations within the existing practice or major renovations that increase the footprint of the office. At the beginning, it is wise to use existing space before considering major alterations to the office. If multiple offices are present, allergy services can also be centralized to the one which is most suitable.

The allergy treatment area is the space where patients will undergo skin testing, counseling, blood testing, allergy injections, and possible pulmonary function testing. While there are no strict requirements for this space, it should be able to accommodate one or more seated patients and the allergy care provider without feeling crowded. An outside window is ideal to create the appearance of more space and promote a feeling of tranquility while patients are undergoing testing and treatment. If there is space for more than one patient, curtains or other partitions must be used to ensure privacy. The room should have a solid floor to minimize the presence of mold, dust and animal dander, a desk for the allergy care provider, and sufficient counter space to comfortably accommodate a computer, two or three treatment boards, and a refrigerator (▶ Fig. 44.1). There should be cabinet storage space above and below the counter for commonly used supplies, and it is also useful to have a larger storage space in a non-patient area for backup. There should be a sink present in the room, as well as room for a floor refrigerator.

In addition to a treatment area, it is ideal to have a small, separate space for vial preparation and antigen dilution. This area can be an inside space, but should have a refrigerator, sink, a moderate amount of counter space, and a lock on the door. This space is useful because vial preparation should be performed by the allergy care provider without any outside distractions, such as phone calls or questions from staff and patients. This ancillary space is also helpful when there are multiple members of the allergy staff, so that one allergy care provider can be giving injections, while another is preparing a vial.

Extra waiting space is also a consideration. Once allergy patients come into the office, they should be promptly brought back to the treatment room for their injection and ready to leave the office within 30 minutes afterward. This certainly would anger a patient who has been waiting for their physician appointment for the past hour, because they may think that other patients are being seen ahead of them. Ideally, there should be a separate entrance for the allergy patients, which will allow them to check in and be brought to a smaller waiting room that is near or adjacent to the treatment area (▶ Fig. 44.2). This area may also be used by patients during their 30-minute waiting period after an allergy injection.

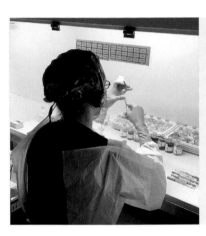

Fig. 44.1 Mixing personnel wearing appropriate garb in a designated area free of distractions.

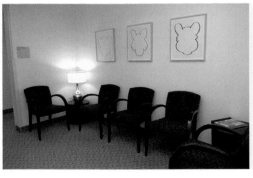

Fig. 44.2 An example of a smaller waiting room for allergy patients.

44.5 Necessary Equipment

44.5.1 Refrigerator

Refrigeration of extracts, testing vials, and immunotherapy vials is helpful to prolong the shelf life of these items. It is helpful to have one larger refrigerator, either free-standing or underneath the counter, which can store the majority of these supplies. None of these supplies need to be frozen, but a freezer may be useful to store ice packs to place on a patient's arm in the event of a large, local reaction. Chemical cold packs, activated by mechanical pressure, are helpful to save space in the refrigerator and can be given to the patient to use even after leaving the office. A small, countertop refrigerator can be helpful to store the items that are used most during the day, such as testing trays. This item will not only spare the back of the allergy care provider from repeated bending and straining, but will also prevent repeated opening and warming of the main supply refrigerator.

44.5.2 Patient Treatment Chair

This should be a comfortable chair, preferably with armrests to provide stability while the patient is undergoing skin testing, receiving an injection, or having blood drawn. A practitioner should look for a chair which will fit both the treatment room as well as the budget. Online supply houses are often used or the retailer can be contacted who has provided other furniture and examination chairs for the office. It may also be helpful to check the local hospital to see if they are discarding any phlebotomy chairs, which may need only minor repairs. This type of chair works very well because it usually has large armrests or a bar that comes down in front to support the arms (▶ Fig. 44.3). Ideally, a treatment chair also has the capability to recline in case a patient develops a vasovagal or anaphylactic reaction, but this type of chair takes up more space.

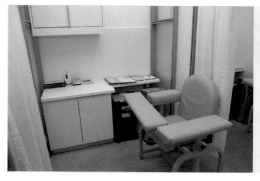

Fig. 44.3 An example of a testing set-up with a chair that has large armrests or a bar that comes down in front to support the arms.

44.5.3 Sharps Containers

These devices are mandated by Occupational Safety and Health Administration (OSHA) and should be installed according to current regulations. One sharps container should be present near each treatment chair and every counter where needles are in use. Skin prick testing devices and discarded vials are also placed in these containers. A large sharps container with wheels may be moved to each area where it is necessary, or smaller ones may be mounted on the walls. Care must also be taken to follow all State and Federal regulations concerning the disposal of sharps containers, which will significantly increase in volume once allergy is added to the practice.

44.5.4 Emergency Kit/Crash Cart

This is a cart or kit containing necessary medications, such as auto-injectable epinephrine, antihistamines, and steroids, as well as laryngoscopes, endotracheal tubes (ETs), and the supplies needed to start an intravenous (IV) line. See Chapter 34 for examples of equipment, medications, and supplies necessary for allergy emergencies and an example of an anaphylaxis protocol. A standard tool chest from the local hardware store or tackle box works perfectly for this (▶ Fig. 44.4). It should have multiple, smaller compartments to store smaller medication vials and drawers for ET tubes, IV tubing, etc. It should be clearly labeled and stored in a place known by all office staff, preferably in the allergy treatment area. It should be checked on a regular basis to make sure that expired medications are re-ordered and batteries for the laryngoscope remain functional. It should also contain medication cards in a small binder to make dose calculations simple in an emergency situation.

Other pieces of equipment required for the treatment of anaphylaxis to be stored in the emergency kit include blood pressure cuffs and stethoscopes. An oxygen tank, preferably on wheels, must be maintained and adequately filled near the allergy treatment area at all times. Oxygen masks and Ambu bags

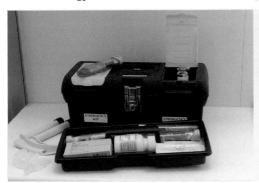

Fig. 44.4 An example of an allergy emergency kit.

should be available along with connecting tubing, suction machine, suction tubing, and suction catheters. You may also consider purchasing an automatic electric defibrillator (AED) for the office.

44.6 Purchasing Supplies

44.6.1 Testing and Treatment Boards

Boards designed to hold 5-mL glass vials are available in a variety of materials, but acrylic works very well for this purpose. They are sturdy and fit well on most small refrigerator racks. They are available with 6 columns across to hold all the dilutions necessary for a particular antigen, and 10 rows deep to hold enough antigens for a particular session of intradermal testing. As a convention, the #6 dilution is on the left side of the board and these numbers should be written on the side of the board with permanent black marker to avoid any confusion. Concentrated antigens are never stored on the testing and treatment boards. The same board may be used for testing and treatment. If multiple antigen treatment vials are prepared for each patient, they should be stored in the refrigerator as well.

44.6.2 Syringes

Three types of syringes are available: (1) testing syringes, (2) treatment syringes, and (3) mixing syringes. Testing syringes have a 3/8-inch short bevel to allow for intradermal injection. They are usually 0.5 mL syringes with a 27-G needle attached, but 1 mL syringes and 26 G needles are also available. Treatment syringes are typically 1 mL in volume with a 26-G, half-inch needle with a longer bevel to enter the subcutaneous space. However, 3/8 inch needles are also available in gauge sizes as small as 28 G. Testing and treatment syringes can also be obtained with a safety feature that allows instant protection of the needle once it is used. Mixing syringes, with a 23-G, half-inch needle are very useful because 1 mL of fluid can be drawn up and released with minimum strain to the fingers. It is difficult to know the quantity of each syringe needed to order in the beginning, but this will become clear in a short time. It is important to use allergy syringes that have integrated needles. Using tuberculin syringes, or other syringes with removable needles, will lead to inaccurate testing and treatment because a small amount of fluid is left in the hub after the plunger is fully depressed.

44.6.3 Skin Prick Testing Devices

These devices are available from most allergy supply houses in both single prick and multiple prick varieties. They are made of disposable plastic and usually contain multiple tines at the end of each arm to hold extract through capillary forces. Concentrated extract may be placed on the skin and the device pricked through the droplet into the epidermis, or the device may be stored in trays containing extract-filled wells. These trays have a sticker on the cover to clearly label which antigen is in each well, and the trays nest with the cover and other trays for easy storage. Trays must always be held by the bottom, not the cover, when transporting them. Each well should be filled with approximately 0.7 mL of concentrated extract. Filling to the top of the well will decrease the time interval for refilling, but may lead to extract overflow and contamination of neighboring wells. Trays should be replaced periodically or when extract residue is present around the wells. In the beginning, it is reasonable to order a large volume of skin prick devices, as this inventory will move quickly. This is particularly true if 2 or 3 units are used for each patient per session.

44.6.4 Allergen Extracts

Concentrated extracts are usually purchased in standardized potency concentrations or as a 1:20 w/v, or weight per volume concentration. This means that 1 g of antigen extract is present in 20 mL of solution. This does not indicate the amount of major antigen in each solution, nor does it guarantee a certain antigenic activity of the extract. Unfortunately, there is still a significant variability in different antigen batches, but if the same allergy supplier is used, this should minimize the variability. Concentrated extracts come in 50% glycerin, which gives them a shelf life of approximately 3 years. Nevertheless, they should be stored in the refrigerator, preferably grouped according to the testing panels to make refilling the wells an easier process. Generally, 10 mL vials of concentrate are ordered, but larger sizes are available if needed (▶ Fig. 44.5). The practitioner must decide which antigens to test and treat with, but at least one or two

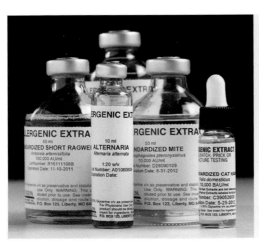

Fig. 44.5 Different size vials of allergen concentrates.

antigens from each major class is appropriate for initial testing. Some antigens, such as dust mite, cat dander, and molds, will be standard in all locations, but tree, grass, and weed pollens will vary depending on the region of the practice.

44.6.5 Glass Vials, With or Without Diluent

Empty, 5 mL glass vials are used for creating a multidose immunotherapy vial. They have a soft membrane at the top with a metal cuff just like other injection vials. Similar vials are also available with 4 mL of diluent present, usually phenolated saline or human serum albumin. These are used for the creation of fivefold dilutions of the concentrated extract for intradermal testing. Usually, 1 mL of extract is mixed with 4 mL of phenolated saline to create a fivefold dilution. The first dilution of the concentrated extract (#1) will have a 10% glycerin concentration, giving it a 3-month shelf life in the refrigerator, while the subsequent dilutions (#2 to #6) will only have a 6-week shelf life.

44.6.6 Diluent, Histamine, and Glycerin

The most common diluent in use today is phenolated saline. This is a buffered, saline solution that is resistant to the growth of bacteria and viruses. It is used in the creation of fivefold dilutions of concentrated extract, as one of the controls used during intradermal testing and to correct the volume of an immunotherapy treatment vial. Some offices also use human serum albumin as a diluent. Aqueous histamine phosphate available at a concentration of 0.275 mg/mL is used. This may be diluted for single intradermal or intradermal dilutional testing. Histamine at a concentration of either 1 mg/mL histamine base (2.75 mg/mL histamine phosphate) or 6 mg/mL histamine base (10 mg/mL histamine dichloride) in a 50% glycerin base is used as a positive control for skin prick testing. Glycerin at a concentration of 50% may be obtained in 100 mL vials and used as the negative control for SPT. Dilutions of this solution (#1 to #3) are used during intradermal dilutional testing because glycerin itself can produce a wheal and flare reaction in certain individuals. The purpose of glycerin is to preserve the shelf life of the solution and it is added to immunotherapy treatment vials to assure at least a 10% glycerin concentration.

44.6.7 Other Supplies

Many of the necessary supplies are already stocked in the office, but will have to be ordered in larger amounts once allergy is added. This includes alcohol pads, markers, labels, timers, ice packs, and topical antihistamine skin spray. Cardboard rulers, with semicircular cutouts to measure wheal sizes, are available from allergy suppliers. Dropper vials and metered-dose pumps for SLIT are available in both glass and plastic (▶ Fig. 44.6). Educational handouts

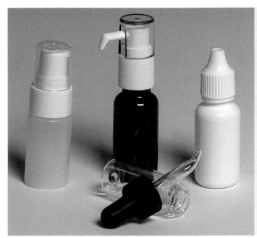

Fig. 44.6 Dropper vials and metered-dose pumps for sublingual immunotherapy (SLIT).

concerning allergic rhinitis, allergen avoidance, and immunotherapy should be prepared for patients to take home, and examples of products, such as dust mite barriers, should also be available for demonstration.

44.7 Documentation

Most offices use electronic medical records as this type of documentation works very well with allergy services. A template should be created in the computer so that prick testing results can be easily entered. It should include the date, ordering physician, person performing the test, site of testing, antigen used, grade, wheal diameter, and space for comments. Likewise, templates for intradermal testing and vial formulation should also be created. It is helpful to create similar paper forms to jot results down while at the patient's side if the computer is not readily available. The immunotherapy record should contain the date, vial number, immunotherapy plan (escalate, decrease, repeat, or maintain), dose, and the diameter of the resulting induration.

In addition to the testing and treatment records, it is important for both physician and allergy care provider to document the extent of all interactions with the allergy patient. After testing, the provider should document all environmental control strategies discussed and the time spent counseling. During an immunotherapy session, the provider must indicate the patient's current symptom state, current medications being used, and any adverse reactions from the previous injection. On some occasions, the provider may provide counseling on an unrelated issue, such as sinusitis or ear pain, and this additional evaluation and management should also be carefully documented. The supervising physician must then review all of the provider's records and notes and document this in the patient's record as well.

Clinical Pearls **M!**

- Consult with partners and practice advisers as soon as the idea of adding allergy to the practice is considered.
- Create a budget and determine whether or not adding allergy to the practice is financially feasible.
- Take courses and obtain the proper training before moving forward.
- Use existing space prior to making any major renovations to the office.
- Choose allergy care providers carefully and supervise closely.
- Start with a few straightforward patients and build the allergy practice slowly.
- Learn how to perform and teach every aspect of allergy testing and treatment.
- Stay actively involved in the allergy practice.

Bibliography

[1] Burton MJ, Krouse JH, Rosenfeld RM. Extracts from The Cochrane Library: Sublingual immunotherapy for allergic rhinitis. Otolaryngol Head Neck Surg. 2011; 144(2):149–153

[2] Houser SM, Keen KJ. The role of allergy and smoking in chronic rhinosinusitis and polyposis. Laryngoscope. 2008; 118(9):1521–1527

[3] Marple BF, Mabry RL. Quantitative Skin Testing for Allergy: IDT and MQT. New York, NY: Thieme; 2006

[4] Noon L. Prophylactic inoculation against hay fever. Lancet. 1911; 1:1572–1573

45 Patient Selection

Cecelia C. Damask

45.1 Putting the Pieces Together

While a presumptive diagnosis of allergic rhinitis (AR) can be made based on history and physical examination, testing for specific immunoglobulin E (IgE) antibodies to inhalant allergen(s) to which the patient reports symptoms helps confirm the diagnosis of AR and allows for potential treatment with immunotherapy. However to do this, several things are needed: a patient with symptoms consistent with allergy, specific allergy tests, and perhaps most importantly, a physician capable of interpreting the test results in light of the patient's symptoms. Only if all of the above items are "checked off the list" is it likely that a correct allergy diagnosis will be made.

45.2 Serious Stuff

Proper evaluation and selection of which patients may benefit from skin testing is crucial.
- Condition and reactivity of the skin can affect skin test results. Avoid skin testing patients with:
  - Dermatographism.
  - Diffuse urticaria.
  - Active dermatitis.
- Proper selection of where the skin tests are to be placed is also important.
  - Skin pricks can be placed on the upper back or volar surface of the forearm.
  - The back is more reactive than the forearms.
  - Intradermals can be placed on upper arm.
  - Regardless of location, there needs to be sufficient space (about 2–2.5 cm) between each allergen applied.
  - Tests should not be placed in areas 5 cm from the wrist or 3 cm from the antecubital fossae.
- Medications could alter the validity of the results. A large range of drugs may reduce skin reactivity and must be withheld before skin testing including:
  - First-generation and second-generation antihistamines
    a) This includes eyedrops and nasal spray preparations.
    b) The duration of suppression of skin test reactivity is variable between different drugs and individuals.
  - Antidepressants such as doxepin and other tricyclics have antihistamine activity.

- Over-the-counter (OTC) preparations such as cold and flu remedies, "sinus" analgesics, antitussives, H2 blockers, etc., can affect skin response.
- Herbal products have the potential to affect skin test results.
- Antiemetics, sedatives, and muscle relaxants can also affect skin response.
- Short-term oral corticosteroids do not significantly diminish the skin test reaction but may with prolonged use.
- Prolonged topical corticosteroids have been shown to reduce skin reactivity.
- Omalizumab can suppress skin reactivity.
- Special class of medication:
  - Beta blockers are a risk factor for more serious and treatment-resistant anaphylaxis, making the use of beta blockers a relative contraindication to inhalant skin testing.
- Relative contraindications/precautions:
  - Poor subject cooperation.
  - Patients unable to cease antihistamines or other medications.
  - Persistent severe/unstable asthma.
  - Pregnancy.

Proper selection of which patients may benefit from immunotherapy is paramount to good outcomes with immunotherapy.

Allergen immunotherapy should be considered for patients who have evidence of specific IgE antibodies to clinically relevant allergens demonstrated either through skin testing or in vitro specific IgE testing. The commitment to begin allergen immunotherapy is a shared decision between the physician and the patient after reviewing the patient's response to medical management, including adverse effects of medications, response to avoidance measures, likelihood of adherence to an immunotherapy schedule, and patient preference. The severity and duration of symptoms along with effect on the patient's quality of life should also be considered when assessing the need to proceed with immunotherapy.

45.3 Precautions to Consider

Relative contraindications/precautions with immunotherapy include:
- Poor subject cooperation/inability to commit to the immunotherapy schedule.
- Unstable asthma.
- Pregnancy.
- Beta blockers are a risk factor for more serious and treatment-resistant anaphylaxis.

Clinical Pearls **M!**

- Proper patient selection is crucial both with skin testing and the provision of immunotherapy.
- Review all the patients' medical conditions including skin pathology such as dermatographism and asthma control prior to skin testing.
- Review all of the patient's medications prior to skin testing.
- Make sure patients are aware of which medications to discontinue prior to skin testing.

Bibliography

[1] Bernstein IL, Li JT, Bernstein DI, et al. American Academy of Allergy, Asthma and Immunology, American College of Allergy, Asthma and Immunology. Allergy diagnostic testing: an updated practice parameter. Ann Allergy Asthma Immunol. 2008; 100(3) Suppl 3:S1–S148

[2] Cox L, Nelson H, Lockey R, et al. Allergen immunotherapy: a practice parameter third update. J Allergy Clin Immunol. 2011; 127(1) Suppl:S1–S55

46 Nurse Selection and Training

William R. Reisacher, Matthew W. Ryan, Cecelia C. Damask

46.1 Hiring Personnel

When adding allergy to the practice, there may be no need to hire new personnel. The allergist should be able to perform all the tasks required and may enjoy the opportunity to utilize their skills. However, as the allergy service becomes busier, additional staff must be recruited to the allergy team to save allergist's time and energy. This should be a person(s) who is qualified to perform the job being asked and has been adequately trained by the allergist, who ultimately is responsible for that person's performance. The physician may train an existing medical assistant or nurse to perform some of the duties, such as skin testing, immunotherapy injections, patient counseling, and inventory. Other duties, such as immunotherapy vial preparation, could be done by a non-care provider who has a background in laboratory work or a pharmacy technician.

In time, most of the duties of a busy allergy service will be in the hands of one or more allergy care providers who will likely be new employees. There may be multiple part-time employees, one full-time employee, or any other combination, but continuity of care from testing and counseling to vial preparation and immunotherapy is an important factor to consider. The allergy staff functions in many ways as a care provider who will likely see the allergy patients much more frequently than the allergist. Patients confide in this person in a way that they would not with the physician. This is why communication between the allergist and allergy care staff is critically important. While the physician will always be directing the allergy care, the allergy care provider should be able to work more independently as experience is gained.

There is no official training program or certification for allergy care providers, but a registered nurse (RN) or licensed practical nurse (LPN) tends to function best in this capacity. It may be possible to find someone who has worked as an allergy care provider before, but they will likely have to undergo some retraining by the allergist because each allergist may have slightly different preferences and methods. Nurses with no prior allergy experience will naturally have to undergo more extensive training. This is why it is so important for the allergist to receive sufficient training, not only to perform all the tasks required, but also to be able to teach the allergy care provider. New graduates from nursing programs may be recruited, but allergy testing and treatment is not part of their standard curriculum, and all this training must be received from the allergist for whom they are working. In addition to advertising in local newspapers and medical journals, courses and meetings are excellent places to network with other allergists and find allergy care providers who may be interested in relocating.

The allergy care provider will be heavily relied upon by the allergist. This person must be easy to work with and have good communication skills. They should be neat, free of strong odors, organized, detail-oriented, and good at multitasking. Good math skills are a plus when it comes to vial formulation and making dilutions of concentrated allergy extracts. When interviewing for the position, the allergist should make sure that the individual is able to perform "hands on" procedures, such as skin testing and venipuncture, but also enjoys interacting with patients. The allergy care provider must understand that they will be following patients over an extended period of time and may frequently be listening to problems that have little to do with allergies. The allergy care provider must also understand that there is a great deal of "on the job" training required. Finally, it is important that the allergy care provider is dependable, because frequent, unplanned absences can be detrimental to both patient care and physician well-being.

While much of the allergy care provider's training will be done by the allergist directly, there are other options as well. Selected chapters in textbooks, such as this one, should be assigned for reading in advance to facilitate the training sessions. It is best to start slowly and build upon fundamental principles. Make a schedule for training sessions with reasonable deadlines for completion. Too much information given at once will only create confusion and frustration for all parties involved. Outside educational opportunities are also available. Many nurses attend continuing medical education (CME) courses with their allergist and other courses are available online or through nursing societies. It is best to create a list of responsibilities for the allergy care provider, which may be checked off once the training is complete. This list may include:

- Skin prick testing (SPT).
- Intradermal testing (ID).
- Modified quantitative testing (MQT).
- Venipuncture.
- Giving a subcutaneous injection.
- Anaphylaxis protocol.
- Performing five-fold dilutions of concentrated allergy extracts.
- Vial formulation and preparation, SCIT as well as SLIT.
- Patient counseling, avoidance strategies, and autoinjectable epinephrine demonstration.
- Performing pulmonary function testing.
- Lecturing at courses/enrolling research patients (academic practices).
- Ordering supplies/billing/scheduling/documentation.

As the allergy department begins to expand, there may be other additions to the staff that become necessary. This might include additional front office staff to assist with check-in and making sure that allergy patients move efficiently through the office. The back office staff may also grow to help manage the increased number of claims that are being processed and to make sure payments are being properly collected. Additional middle staff, such as medical assistants, may also be required to take vital signs and assist the allergy care provider with phone calls and inventory. Conversely, the practice may choose to invest in additional technology, such as key fobs so that patients may scan or swipe to check in, text messaging appointment reminders, and electronic payment programs. While the additional employees or technology may not be a part of the initial budget, they must be factored into future budget calculations for the allergy service.

Clinical Pearls   M!

- Pleasant, well-trained allergy care providers are vital to the success of any allergy practice.
- Training should be provided by the allergist in charge.
- There are many opportunities for additional education and training of staff, including live course, textbooks, and online modules.

47 Billing and Coding

Cecelia C. Damask, Matthew W. Ryan, William R. Reisacher

47.1 Most Important Information

Each physician or advanced practice provider is responsible for his/her own coding practices and accuracy. This chapter contains a guide of commonly used allergy Current Procedural Terminology (CPT) codes that are current as of publication, but may change with future revisions of CPT code terminology after this book is published. Be sure to verify with the most current CPT publications to ensure coding accuracy.

47.2 Billing and Coding

When adding allergy to a new or existing practice, the allergist should meet with the billing office staff and explain all the new procedure codes they will be encountering. It may be necessary to add billing staff to accommodate the increase in claims volume or update any billing/coding or electronic medical record software. Insurance companies should also be contacted so that fee schedules and covered services are spelled out clearly and obtained in writing. Most of the procedures billed by the allergy care provider are "incident to" services and are paid under the physician's fee schedule. An "incident to" service must be part of the patient's normal course of treatment. The physician must have performed the initial service and must remain actively involved in the treatment course. Although the physician does not have to be in the room where the service is performed, he or she must be in the immediate area providing direct supervision. This must also be clearly stated in the patient's record. The most common CPT® codes used for allergy services are discussed further.

95004: This code is used for skin prick testing for airborne or food allergens. The number of units assigned to this code corresponds to the number of antigens and controls tested. The reporting of the results and the interpretation by the physician is included in this code.

If a prick test was performed using 10 antigens plus the positive and negative controls, 95004 would be billed for 12 units.

95024: This code is used for intradermal testing when a single dilution of an allergen or control is tested, with the number of units corresponding to the number of tests placed. Again, interpretation and reporting are included in this code. When skin prick testing is done at the same time as intradermal testing, 95004 may be billed at the same time as the intradermal codes.

95027: This code is used for intradermal testing when multiple dilutions of an allergen or control are tested, with the number of units corresponding to the total number of tests placed, including interpretation and reporting. Certain insurance companies do not reimburse 95027 and the billing staff should keep track of this to avoid a claim being denied.

> If intradermal dilutional testing was performed using 2 antigens where 4 dilutions each were placed, 95027 would be billed for 8 units.

95115: This code is used when one immunotherapy injection is given and does not include the provision of allergy extracts. No units are assigned to this code.

95117: This code is the same as 95115, except that more than one immunotherapy injection is given. These codes (95115 and 95117) can never be billed together. There are no units assigned to this code.

95165: This code covers the professional services for supervising and preparing an immunotherapy vial. It is billed as soon as the vial is prepared, usually on a day when the patient is not in the office and no other testing or treatment services are being provided. For a 5-mL vial, the number of units depends on the "billable" dose. Although a "treatable" dose may be 0.5 mL, Medicare and some other insurance companies use 1 mL as a "billable" dose, and therefore 5 units would be billed for this service. Other insurance companies allow 0.5 mL as a "billable" dose, and for these claims, 10 units may be billed. The billing staff should check with each carrier to clarify their specific policies.

47.3 Supervision Requirements

Medicare requires direct physician supervision of allergy testing services. Allergy diagnostic skin testing services are to be reported using the on-site supervising physician's name and National Provide Number (NPI) number. Advanced practice providers (APPs) (such as physician assistants and nurse practitioners) may not bill for supervised skin testing. APPs may bill using their own NPI for any testing they personally perform but they can't supervise a nurse or a technician performing the allergy test. Requirements concerning who may bill for allergy services, and at which level, varies from state to state, so it is prudent to clarify the details in the state where you practice.

Medicare also requires direct physician or other qualified health care provider supervision of allergy immunotherapy including injections and vial preparation. The service is reported using the on-site supervising provider's name and NPI number. The date of service for the charge for vial preparation (95165) is the date that the vial was mixed and it should be billed using the on-site provider's name and NPI number. As per the Medicare requirements, these services cannot be billed under a physician who is not physically in the office (i.e., a surgeon in the operating room) when the service is performed.

Clinical Pearls

- Be sure to discuss/educate billing staff on CPT codes they will see when adding/starting an allergy practice.
- Allergy services are "incident to," meaning a provider does not have to be directly in the testing/treatment room, but must be in the immediate office suite. This includes billing for vial mixing/preparation services as well.
- Testing CPT codes are billed by the number of units/tests placed and include controls.
- Injection codes do not include units.
- Injection vials may be billed either by number of "billable" 1 mL doses, or by "treatable" doses. Be sure to check with each insurer so that billing staff are accurate when submitting claims.

Index

A

AAP *see* American Academy of Pediatrics (AAP)
acupuncture 136
AD *see* atopic dermatitis (AD)
adaptive immune response 2
adaptive immune system 2
adaptive immunity 2
add allergy 252
aeroallergen 6
age-related (senile) rhinitis 48
airway hyperresponsiveness 194
allergen, extract 248, 261
allergen 15
allergen immunotherapy 266
allergenic grasses 20
allergenic molds 27
allergenic pollens 18
allergenic trees, types of 22
allergenic trees 23
allergenic weeds 32, 34
allergic disorders 126
allergic inflammation 13
allergic reactions 177
allergic rhinitis
– classification system 6
– definition 6
– severity 8
allergic rhinitis 48, 113, 117, 122
Allergic Rhinitis in Asthma (ARIA) guidelines 6
allergic shiner *46*
allergic-contact dermatitis 202
allergy
– injections 146
– medications 107
– symptoms 38
– testing *73*
– testing syringe *72*
– toothpaste 165
allergy 9
allergy care provider 269
allergy emergency kit *259*
allergy training 254

allergy, preparing space for 256
alternaria 27
alternative remedies 135
amaranth-chenopods 33
amaranthaceae family 33, 35
amaranths 36
American Academy of Pediatrics (AAP) 200
ammi visnaga 119
amphiphilous 17
anaphylaxis
– kit *179*
– protocol 181
– signs and symptoms of 180
– strikes 180
anaphylaxis 58, 176
anemophilus 17
angiosperms, trees 22–24
angiosperms 18, 35
anthemideae (sage) tribe 32
anti-human IgE antibody 89
anticholinergics 105
antigen 15
antigen dilutions 70
antigen presenting cells (APCs) 3
antigens test 71
antihistamine–decongestant combinations 104
antihistamines 107
APCs *see* antigen presenting cells (APCs)
aqueous histamine 77
aqueous histamine phosphate 262
aqueous sublingual immunotherapy vial 154
ARIA guidelines *see* Allergic Rhinitis in Asthma (ARIA) guidelines
ascomycota 26
aseptic compounding technique, measure 250
aseptic compounding technique 249
asteraceae family 32, 35
asthma
– control 195

– of future 198
asthma 52, 126, 194
asthma exacerbation 185
atopic dermatitis (AD) 126, 210

B

B-cells, survival 131
B-cells 3
baccharis species 33
Bahia grass 19
balloon Sinuplasty 164
basidiomycota phylum 26
basophils 4
BAU *see* bioequivalent allergy unit (BAU)
benralizumab 131
Bermuda grass pollen 19
beta-blockers 55
billing 271
bioequivalent allergy unit (BAU) 16
biologics 126
black box warning 118
blended techniques 84
bluish discoloration of mucosa *46*
brassicaceae 35
bronchoconstriction 115, 194
buoyant pollen 22
butterbur 137

C

cannabaceae family 34–35
cannibalism 164
cat antigens 30
caution 102
cellular differentiation 131
cereal grains 19
chemical rhinitis 49
chenopod family 33, 36
chenopodiaceae family 35
chronic idiopathic urticaria (CIU) 126
cichorieae tribe 33

Index

grass
- allergens 18
- pollen 15
grass pollen antigens 18
grastek 161
gymnosperm, trees 22, 24
gymnosperms 18

H

hands on procedures 269
HDM *see* house dust mites (HDM)
headache 48
heliantheae tribe 32, 36
herbal remedies 137
herbal therapies 136
heterogeneous disorder 210
high-dose immunotherapy 147
hiring personnel 268
histamines
- control 77
- H1 107
- H2 107
- types of *58*
histamines 107, 262
history of present illness (HPI) 38
honey 135
hormonal rhinitis 49
house dust mite (HDM) 98, 162
HPI *see* history of present illness (HPI)
humanized monoclonal anti-IL-5 antibody 131
hypersensitivity reactions 2
hypoallergenic pets 30

I

IDT technique *see* intradermal dilutional testing (IDT) technique
IgE-mediated reactions 202
immediate reactions 184
immune system
- bias 4
- simplification of 4
immunoglobulin E (IgE)

- benralizumab 131
- dupilumab 132
- interleukin-4 and interleukin-13 132
- interleukin-5 131
- librikizumab and tralokinumab 132
- mepolizumab 131
- omalizumab 126
- reslizumab 131
- tezepelumab 133
- thymic stromal lymphopoietin 132
immunoglobulin E (IgE) 88
immunoglobulins 3
immunology
- adaptive immune responses 2
- adaptive immunity 2
- hypersensitivity reactions 2
- immune system, simplification of 4
- major players 3
- tolerance and immune system bias 4
immunotherapy 92, 139, 150, 255
imposters 48
in vitro allergy testing 90
inflammatory condition of nasal mucosa 6
inhalant allergen, allergenic pollens 18
inhalant allergens
- allergenic grasses 20
- allergenic molds 27
- allergenic trees, types of 22
- allergenic trees 23
- allergenic weeds 32, 34
- antigen and allergen 15
- cross-reactivity 16
- dust and danders 29
- grass allergens 18
- grasses pollinate 19
- major allergenic trees 25
- major allergens 27, 30, 36
- minor families 34
- mold allergy 26
- nonstandardized allergen extracts 16

- pet dander 30
- pollen 18
- spores 26
- springtime tree troubles 22
- standard allergen extracts 25, 28, 31, 36
- standardized allergen extracts 16
- Thommen's postulates 17
- trees pollinate 23
- weeds
-- imposters 32
-- pollinate 34
- weeds 32
inhalant allergy, specific immunoglobulin E testing for 88
injectable corticosteroid preparations 113
injection escalation protocols 147
innate immune system 2
interleukin
- 4 132
- 5 131
- 13 132
- 31, nemolizumab 133
intermittent symptoms 7
intradermal dilutional testing (IDT) technique 81
intradermal dilutional testing case 221–222
intradermal dilutional testing vial mixing case version 1 228–229
intradermal dilutional testing vial mixing case version 2 230–231
intradermal testing, for penicillin allergy *191*
intradermal testing 69, 190
intramuscular injections 113
intranasal antihistamines 108
intranasal corticosteroids 111–113
intranasal decongestants 102–103
irritant rhinitis 49
isolated urticaria 186